SIMPLE GIFTS

SIMPLE GIFTS

MEMOIRS OF A HOMETOWN DOCTOR

Harold S. Jenkins, M.D.

Copyright © 2015 by Doreen Jenkins.

Library of Congress Control Number:		2015918851
ISBN:	Hardcover	978-1-5144-1673-0
	Softcover	978-1-5144-1771-3
	eBook	978-1-5144-1672-3

All rights reserved. No part of this book may be reproduced or transmitted in any form or by any means, electronic or mechanical, including photocopying, recording, or by any information storage and retrieval system, without permission in writing from the copyright owner.

Any people depicted in stock imagery provided by Thinkstock are models, and such images are being used for illustrative purposes only.
Certain stock imagery © Thinkstock.

Print information available on the last page.

Rev. date: 02/23/2016

To order additional copies of this book, contact:
Xlibris
1-888-795-4274
www.Xlibris.com
Orders@Xlibris.com
719351

CONTENTS

Preface ix

Chapter One: The Exam Room Quartet 1

Chapter Two: A House Call At Hebron Hill 7

Chapter Three: My Mother's Crystal Ball 13

Chapter Four: The Sketch In The Chestnut Frame 19

Chapter Five: Coronary Angioplasty And Barley Green Tea 26

Chapter Six: On Sedatives And Church Attendance 33

Chapter Seven: The Octopus's Asthma Attack 39

Chapter Eight: Mrs. Marshall's Surprise 45

Chapter Nine: An Office Christmas Eve With Jimmy 51

Chapter Ten: A Diet Plan For Mrs. Holmes 58

Chapter Eleven: The Crayon Drawing 64

Chapter Twelve: Health-Care Delivery By Bulldozer 71

Chapter Thirteen: Heartbreak On Walker's Bottom Road 78

Chapter Fourteen: Old Knees And Older Animosities 84

Chapter Fifteen: Ella Mae Blossom Goes To Staunton 90

Chapter Sixteen: The Knock On The Door 96

Chapter Seventeen: Mrs. Simpson Attacks Pornography 103

Chapter Eighteen: Cholesterol Screening And Sausage Gravy 110

Chapter Nineteen: Reverend Detamore Steps Over The Line 117

Chapter Twenty: Mrs. Middlebrook's Revolver 123

Chapter Twenty-One: A Man's Tears 129

Chapter Twenty-Two: Dark Secret On Main Street 136

Chapter Twenty-Three: Mrs. Mcallister's Top Priority 142

Chapter Twenty-Four: The Photograph Cure 149

Chapter Twenty-Five: A Miser And A Lover 154

Chapter Twenty-Six: A Midnight Caller 159

Chapter Twenty-Seven: The Chocolate Cake Cure 165

Chapter Twenty-Eight: Public Relations, Here I Come! 170

Chapter Twenty-Nine: A Day In The Life Of A Medical Movie Star 176

Chapter Thirty: Mr. Wenger's Last Poem 182

'Tis a gift to be simple,
'Tis a gift to be free,
'Tis a gift to come down where you ought to be.
And when we find ourselves in the place just right,
'T'will be in the valley of love and delight.

—The Shaker Hymn Book

PREFACE

> **People are constantly trying to use you to help them create the particular illusions by which they live . . . You must not allow yourself to be represented as someone in whom a few of the favorite daydreams of the public have come true.**
> —Thomas Merton, *Conjectures*

In 1985, I joined the Bengal tiger and the whooping crane on the list of endangered species: I became one of the handful of contemporary American physicians who actually opened medical offices in their small hometowns.

For me, this was Madison County, Virginia, a pastoral Blue Ridge Mountain community of long-established farmers and fruit growers. Separated from Washington, D.C., by eighty-five miles and by two centuries of sharp cultural difference, Madison has its reasons for being wary of the nearby national government.

During the Civil War, the local population—thoroughly ambivalent in its allegiance to the Confederacy—was nevertheless devastated by the clash of marauding rival armies. Still recovering in 1930, Madison saw the Western sixth of its area forcibly annexed by the creation of the Shenandoah National Park, an action that evicted two hundred area families from their homesteads.

As dutiful Madison County citizens, my parents passed on to me their unshakable theology about the Civil War in which three of my great-grandfathers had been soldiers. They also joined a chorus of extended relatives—forty aunts and uncles and an uncounted roster of cousins—in denouncing the national park, which had seized all but a fraction of my grandfather's farm.

As the first medical doctor to evolve from a long line of apple growers, I was destined to walk a somewhat different road. In my four years at the University of Virginia Medical School, I listened to my professors with their often contradictory views of health-care delivery. While publicly acknowledging that nearby rural communities needed family doctors, they privately steered their students toward greener pastures.

By 1985, I had completed my residency in emergency medicine and had six years of satisfying hospital experience under my belt. As the father of four energetic children, I surprised even my wife, Doreen, by agreeing to move back to my hometown to begin a family practice. I would be replacing Madison's veteran physician, Dr. Alma Rucker, who had retired to Arizona.

When I left my hometown for college twenty years before, I had been a gangly farm boy. Now, after a most improbable metamorphosis, I was returning as the "new doctor." For neighbors and friends who had known me as a teenager, my reincarnation was difficult to accept. And since I chose to walk in the shining footsteps of my revered predecessor, I quickly came to recognize—and chafe under—the power of precedent.

With startling rapidity, two powerful forces dominated my reentry onto the back roads of Madison County. In my new venture, I first discovered that there were no established boundary markers to guide the novice native doctor. Dr. Rucker, originally from New York City and always an unmarried woman, had been completely dedicated to her loyal army of patients. Her twenty-four-hour availability was the stuff of local legend. In introducing newer and more expensive medical methods, I faced a skeptical audience that of necessity included dozens of my relatives and high school friends. Every day, I found myself wrestling with the explosive issue of personal and professional boundaries.

In my new medical practice, I also soon identified a second force, more subtle but equally potent: the moments of honest personal contact that joined me to my patients. Far away from the high-tech treadmill of the emergency department, my office exam room became the stage for the sharing of a variety of simple gifts. In my Aunt Lillian's still-warm-from-the-oven lemon pound cake or in a child's colorful crayon drawing resided the vitality of the personal touch—a power in human well-being that has been overlooked by the arrogant bureaucrats of managed health care.

Simple Gifts

In this book of authentic stories (with numerous details altered to protect patient confidentiality), I offer a glimpse backward toward a time that may already be extinct—to an era when professional boundary lines were still electric with controversy and when a mutual exchange of simple gifts offered fresh courage to both physicians and their patients.

CHAPTER ONE

THE EXAM ROOM QUARTET

> And malt does more than Milton can
> To justify God's ways to man.
> Ale, man, ale's the stuff to drink
> For fellows whom it hurts to think.
> —A. E. Housman, *A Shropshire Lad*

"Can you sign this, Dr. Jenkins?" Resplendent in fluorescent orange coveralls, a burly paramedic completely filled the doorway of my windowless cubicle. In our new medical office, this renovated closet was my private retreat. "This is the run sheet on the patient I called you about."

Reaching for the paperwork, I glanced first at my visitor's bronzed nametag—Rob Thorson, Paramedic—and then at the rough lumber stacked against the unpainted plasterboard. Our remodeling project, like most things in my native county, was moving along at a barely detectable speed. "It sounds like you've had a busy day," I said to the giant man.

When the paramedic nodded, he looked like an unconcerned modern-day Atlas eager to hoist the world onto his massive shoulders. "Oh, it was going all right until Uncle Fred smashed his car into the garage wall. He's got a fair-sized gash on his head, but otherwise, I think he's okay."

"How did it happen?"

"Just like it did last month, Doc!" When Rob grinned, white teeth flashed from the center of a curly black beard. "Now and again, Uncle Fred drinks a little, and sometimes he can't maneuver that big Buick through the garage door. Last month, he just bumped his head, and I didn't take him anywhere. This time I figure he needs a few stitches."

I looked at the run sheet: November 12, 1985. Motor vehicle accident, Madison, Virginia. Fred H. Thorson Sr.

Quickly, I glanced up. "Rob, is this the Mr. Thorson who used to teach math at the high school?"

"Sure is, Doc. Uncle Fred taught there for over forty years. Aunt Lottie died just this past summer—cancer, you know." Rob picked up the yellow copy of the run sheet. "I'll take him back home when you're finished, Doc. I'm certainly glad that you've opened your new office here in Madison."

As Rob ambled back to the waiting room, I stared at my pink copy of the run sheet. The masculine scrawl was entirely too legible. In my fledgling medical office, at this very moment, my high school algebra teacher had arrived and was awaiting my assistance.

Walking into the solitude of the lab, I gazed through the window into the advancing autumn twilight. Twenty years ago, I had graduated from the small rural high school just two miles up the road. Now the weight of the intervening decades pressed down on me as I recalled my less-than-stellar performance in that long-ago algebra class.

Never a good math student, I had signed up for algebra only because it was a college entrance requirement. My approach was simple enough—I would memorize the sample problems and then mindlessly replicate them on tests.

As methods go, it had not been foolproof. Even when I arrived at a correct answer, Mr. Thorson was undeceived by the thin veneer of my performance and could sense that I had only the haziest idea of what was going on. In uneasy joint sessions at the chalkboard, he would demonstrate for me the lofty superiority of his logical method. Then he would return me to my seat with the admonition to stop memorizing problems and to study the process of logic.

At the end of my first year in Mr. Thorson's class, I was grateful for my B minus. And although after twenty years of medical practice I am still searching for a single practical use for algebra, I have found Mr. Thorson's systematic method to be unfailingly helpful.

From the adjacent exam room came the energetic tinkle and clatter of medical instruments. My nurse, Ellen, was setting up a surgical tray. I had first met Ellen when we were both in high school, but I had worked with her for only a few weeks. Before she and her dairy farmer husband produced their two children, Ellen had been an emergency department nurse, and our ideas of office efficiency were an excellent fit. Already, I knew that this vivacious assistant was invaluable.

"Dr. Jenkins, we're ready." Ellen's crisp summons shattered my reverie. Taking a twenty-year leap forward in time, I carefully buttoned up my starched lab coat. Stepping over the pile of lumber, I strode down the hall and hoped for a briskly effective entrance.

"Hello, Mr. Thorson!" I said.

From under the paper sheet, the figure on the exam table extended a firm handshake. "Hello, Harold. It's been a long time."

Mr. Thorson's voice still resonated with authority, but his face was more wrinkled, and his iron gray hair was thinner. Over the years, his nose had grown larger and redder. It had also acquired a telltale network of tiny purple veins, which suggested a miniature map to area liquor stores. Floating around the exam table was the unmistakable aroma of whiskey.

Ellen's chart note told me that my former teacher took no regular medicines and had already received his tetanus shot. Mr. Thorson recounted that he had been driving into his brick garage and had struck the doorframe. He had been wearing his seat belt and had not lost consciousness. Other than a slight headache, he now felt fine.

A quick physical exam confirmed that Mr. Thorson's injuries were limited to a three-centimeter laceration on his left forehead and a large abrasion over his left temple. The laceration was basically a straight line that should heal reasonably well. The abrasion, however, was an ugly collection of irregular skin tears that looked like a shattered windshield.

I explained to Mr. Thorson that it would probably be harder to get a cosmetically acceptable healing of the abrasion than of the laceration. He nodded. Although he obviously had hit his head with considerable force, there was no evidence of serious internal injury.

Always the efficient medical assistant, Ellen carried on a continuing conversation while I cleaned the skin injuries with Betadine, injected Xylocaine, and clipped off the multiple devitalized edges of the skin tears. Mr. Thorson's laceration was deeper than I had suspected; its closure required two layers of sutures.

Mr. Thorson, it turned out, was now living by himself. His only descendant, Fred Jr., managed a computer software firm in California. Mr. Thorson got to see his two grandchildren twice a year—in the summertime, they spent a week in Madison, and at Christmas, Mr. Thorson flew to Los Angeles. He talked to them on the phone every two weeks.

Since his wife's death, Mr. Thorson did all of his own housework, including cooking. With only rudimentary culinary skills, he limited his excursions to the local supermarket, and in fact, he mostly stayed home. With his declining eyesight, his attraction to science fiction novels had faded.

"Well, we're all through for today," I announced, peeling off the drape.

Tucking back a thick wave of jet-black hair, Ellen nodded. We were both pleased with my handiwork. The laceration had closed into a neat slightly elevated line, and the abrasion had no ragged edges.

Glancing into the wall mirror, Mr. Thorson added his approval. "Looks like you've done good work, Harold."

I squared my shoulders. Something in my old teacher's tone suggested that while he had assigned me a B minus in algebra, he had just rated me an A plus in office surgery.

When Mr. Thorson sat up, he was a little wobbly; but with Ellen's sturdy guidance, he successfully negotiated the trek around the construction litter and back to the waiting room. He agreed to return in two days for a dressing change.

Before meeting Mr. Thorson again, I mulled over a suitable approach to his underlying problem. Alcoholism is rampant everywhere, even in the quiet backwaters of Madison County. Reflecting on my first three weeks of hometown practice, I thought about the teenage basketball player with the DWI citation, the depressed attorney whose chronic fatigue led to a surprising diagnosis of cirrhosis, and the minister's wife whose secret drinking both enraged and controlled her husband.

In preparing for a professional attack on alcoholism, I always face two daunting dilemmas: I must first pry the lid from an individual's best-kept personal secret and then convince him that a serious medical problem actually exists. If I can break through these formidable roadblocks, then I can nudge my patient toward creative ways of coping with an enemy that is an enigmatic blend of physical disease, emotional hunger, and personal habit.

And for Mr. Thorson, there were additional complications. He was elderly, lived alone, and had few outside contacts. When senior citizens turn to liquor, they often are very reluctant to give up one of the few pleasures that remain in their increasingly narrow lives.

But this time, I decided, the outcome would be different. Mr. Thorson was such a renowned champion of logic that I felt certain that given a carefully constructed argument, he would respond appropriately. When he arrived for his recheck, I had rehearsed my lines, and I was ready.

"Mr. Thorson, your face is healing much more quickly than I would have thought." In fact, the reddened circle of abraded skin was clean and had no drainage. The laceration also looked good, and now that forty-eight hours had passed, the major risk of infection was over.

As I dressed his wounds, I noticed how professional and accommodating Mr. Thorson was in his wingtip shoes and paisley tie. Certainly, he agreed. It would be no problem for him to return next Friday for suture removal. He would also be glad to change his bandage every day.

Looking down at my watch, I paused for a moment to mobilize all my personal willpower. "And now, Mr. Thorson, we need to talk about alcohol and how it's damaging your health."

With one simple sentence, I had destroyed—beyond all hope of reconstruction—my established relationship with my algebra teacher. As a physician, I had uttered a social taboo, had leaped over Mr. Thorson's personal boundary fence, and was trespassing on his life. On some deep inner level, I felt a huge sense of relief. There was no turning back.

Raising snowy patrician eyebrows, Mr. Thorson looked mildly surprised as if he had encountered a regrettable but unforeseen breach of conventional Southern etiquette. "I'm not here to discuss my personal habits, Harold. Alcohol isn't a problem for me like most people. I just drink to relax."

Confronting the reprimand on his familiar forehead, I advanced my presentation as systematically as I could. "Well, let's talk about it anyhow."

And we did. In an awkward but eminently civil conversation, we both seemed to sense that instead of a duo, there was really a quartet in the room—the teacher, the student, the patient, and the doctor. In this unexpected crowd, everyone felt the jolts of sudden role reversals, but when it was all over, we had had a good talk.

Mr. Thorson at this time did not want any medical intervention for his alcohol usage. Still, he accepted information about Alcoholics Anonymous, complete with a local telephone number. When I pointed out the correlation between his drinking and his recent accidents, he seemed skeptical but thoughtful. Standing to leave, he amiably shook my hand and promised to consider my recommendations before his next appointment.

Three days later when I reexamined my patient, I was pleased. The laceration demonstrated excellent apposition, and islands of new pink skin were colonizing the abrasion. Congratulating Mr. Thorson on the effectiveness of his dressing changes, I removed his skin sutures.

"Harold," announced Mr. Thorson with the same self-assured authority that he had always displayed in his algebra classes, "I've thought about our conversation last time." He paused to give me a meaningful look. "Actually, I've thought about it a lot."

I smiled. "I'm glad to hear it."

"And beyond that, I've already made some changes—changes that I feel good about."

Soaring up in my chest was a warm geyser of personal fulfillment. In this golden moment, I knew with complete clarity why I had left the emergency department and had opened a family medicine office in my hometown. Here, standing in front of me, was a patient whose life had been transformed by my professional intervention. In my inner space, the A plus doctor winked his congratulations to the B minus algebra student.

"Have you been able to stop drinking altogether yet, Mr. Thorson?" I basked in the anticipation of his likely response.

"Well, actually, no. I still feel that most of the time, my drinking is not a problem for me—or for anyone else." Mr. Thorson awarded me a professorial glance, and my geyser fizzled.

"Well, tell me about the changes you did make." I managed. With the exam room spinning around me, I seemed once more to be standing—confused and sweaty—in front of a towering chalkboard.

In Mr. Thorson's eyes, a faint twinkle glimmered and then was just as quickly gone.

"Harold, I've already told you that I was drinking on both evenings when I ran into my garage door, and certainly, it was reasonable for you to suggest that I change that behavior. So I thought about my options and realized that putting my car inside the garage is a completely unnecessary habit. Now I just park on the driveway outside. That's a logical behavioral change, and I thank you for bringing it to my attention."

"Well, you're . . . you're certainly welcome," I replied, searching for any response that might be hidden in the bombed-out rubble of my professional self-image. "I do hope that everything goes well for you."

As he buttoned his long khaki topcoat, Mr. Thorson laughed confidently. "I know it will, Harold. It always does when a person lives logically."

CHAPTER TWO

A HOUSE CALL AT HEBRON HILL

The biggest disease today is not leprosy or tuberculosis, but rather the feeling of being unwanted, uncared for and deserted by everybody.
—Mother Teresa, in *The Observer*, October 3, 1971

It was the steepest driveway that I had ever seen. As my Ford pickup turned off the gravel country road, I was glad that the early November rain had not yet changed to what the weatherman was predicting—the first snow of the season.

I glanced at the mailbox; the inscription "Hebron Hill" was partially hidden by sprays of red and yellow bittersweet berries. When I shifted into low gear, my truck gave a protesting jerk.

"Oh, that's all right, old fella." I patted the worn dashboard. "We can make it!" Slowly and cautiously, I climbed the boxwood-lined lane and stopped in front of a spacious brick residence.

This house call would be my first to Hebron Hill. Only this afternoon, Ellen had told me about Ralph Tayson, an elderly stroke patient with a troublesome rash. Dr. Alma Rucker, my professional predecessor in Madison, had routinely made house calls to care for Mr. Tayson's medical needs. Now it was my turn.

Stepping out of my truck, I paused for a moment to appreciate the pastoral vista that in the twilight stretched out like a giant Impressionist canvas. At the foot of Hebron Hill, Black Angus cattle grazed in clover pastures that swept up the river valley to the wooded foothills of the Blue Ridge. On one of those foothill farms, I had spent the first eighteen years of my life.

Picking up my leather medical bag, I carefully walked up the slippery flagstone walkway. Freshly mulched English tea roses bordered the walk. Their scattered pink buds were plaintive reminders of a lost Southern summer.

I climbed the steps and rang the doorbell.

Almost immediately, the solid oak door swung inward, and a husky but friendly voice said, "Dr. Jenkins, come right in. I'm Catherine Lewis."

Hanging my parka on a polished coatrack, I adjusted first to the brightness of the hall chandelier and then to the presence of Mrs. Lewis. Although she was no more than five feet two inches and was in her late seventies, Mrs. Lewis was a *femme formidable.* Carmine lipstick and darkly etched eyebrows accentuated a facial expression of unquestioned self-assurance. Her tailored tweed skirt complemented a carefully pleated white blouse. Powdered cheeks, pearl earrings, and immaculate blue-gray hair softened her military erectness only slightly. As she greeted me, she emanated a faint suggestion of perfume and cigarette smoke.

"I do really appreciate your coming to see my brother, Ralph," Mrs. Lewis said. "Dr. Rucker was always so good about visiting him, and when she retired, I had no idea what we would do next. And now you are going to be Ralph's new doctor."

As she led me into an elegant living room, my hostess shook her head sadly before adding that I would have a hard time living up to the reputation of Dr. Rucker. Reflecting on the whirlwind pace of my first month in Madison, I reluctantly agreed with her sentiments.

"Of course, I'll have to tell you Ralph's history before you see him," said Mrs. Lewis. With a wave, she directed me toward a carved cherry rocker and then chose for herself a rose brocade armchair. "He hasn't talked much since his stroke five years ago."

I nodded, put my medical bag on the oriental carpet, and recalled the thundering ridicule of house calls that had reverberated through medical school lectures. "Every house call is a waste of the doctor's valuable time," Professor Matheson had warned, and in my own experience, I knew that he was on target. In prophesying the doom of rural family practice, Professor Matheson had always been certain that he was right.

But as I felt the pleasant firmness of the rocker panels pressing into my back, I wasn't particularly concerned about Professor Matheson. Below the Delft tiles of the mantel, a wood fire crackled and gleamed, and on a rainy evening, its warmth and glow were seductive. After a long day, it felt good to sit.

"I appreciate your help," I said, settling into the rocker. When providing an initial medical history for a patient, family members usually ramble surprisingly far afield. The pertinent facts—like Easter eggs hidden in an English garden maze—are left for the doctor to discover.

In the emergency department where I had worked for the last six years, we physicians communicated with our patients in speech that was often terse or even telegraphic. Hebron Hill, however, was cut off from my professional past by many cultural miles. Better to make peace with a lost half-hour, I decided, than to try to rush someone like Mrs. Lewis.

My hostess smiled and adjusted herself into her own chair. "Ralph has never been the same since his stroke. He can't talk, and he uses his wheelchair to get around the house."

"Has Ralph been with you for a long time?"

"Ever since my husband died twelve years ago." Mrs. Lewis noted that Ralph at age eighty-one was her only surviving brother. Leaning over to tend the fire, she arched her magnificent eyebrows. "Even though I'm seventy-seven, I'm the youngest member of the family."

She laughed, and then she sighed.

What a different world this is from the emergency department, I thought as my hostess launched into an intricate personal and medical history of Ralph. As an Indiana farm boy, he had fallen out of a pear tree and broken his arm. In World War II, he had sustained a minor shoulder injury. Two years ago, he had developed pneumonia but hadn't been hospitalized because Dr. Rucker, that unfailing medical paragon, had guided him to complete recovery with twice-daily penicillin injections. Ralph didn't enjoy reading, had no hobbies, and mostly just watched TV.

Far away from the storm-tossed waves of emergency medicine, I rode like a surfer on the slowly incoming tide of Mrs. Lewis's narrative. Soothed by the gentle rhythm of the rocker and the flickering light from the fireplace, I had enjoyed watching my hostess's face with its interplay of feelings—empathy, concern, regret, amusement, and cynicism.

But as I listened to the ticking of the antique mantel clock and to the tapping of the rain against the windows, I found myself thinking about that one-of-a-kind driveway. Had it iced over yet?

I was also beginning to think longingly of my delayed dinner. From some inner sanctum, the pleasant spicy smell of baked apples had made its way into the living room. Yes, I reassured myself, now must be the time to focus on the reason for this house call.

"So what can you tell me about Ralph's rash?"

"Oh, his rash! That is why I asked you to come, isn't it?" Dr. Rucker had surmised that the rash, which tended to come and go, was probably caused by some unknown allergy. Moisturizing creams usually helped, but when Ralph had a major flare, Dr. Rucker always cured him with shots.

"Well, come and see for yourself, Dr. Jenkins." With the elastic bound of an Olympic gymnast, Mrs. Lewis stood and nodded toward a nearby doorway. Walking through a solarium fragrant with blossoming orchids, we entered a room where there was a very loud TV.

"Ralph's been a little deaf since his stroke!" shouted Mrs. Lewis in a futile attempt to overpower a blaring football game. Walking up behind the frail man in the wheelchair, she cupped her mouth to his left ear and announced with the intensity of a trumpet fanfare. "Ralph! The new doctor is here!"

A golden Labrador retriever harked a hearty welcome, but his master didn't notice our intrusion until with sisterly authority Mrs. Lewis switched off the TV. As my new patient glanced at me, I jacked up my voice by several decibels. "How are you, Mr. Tayson?"

In complete silence, Ralph offered me a weak left-sided handshake. Across the blue and white checkerboard of his flannel pajamas, his withered right hand lay idle as helpless as a flower blighted by an early frost.

Continuing my fortissimo monologue, I examined Ralph. His rash—red scaling splotches on his forehead, upper chest, and shoulders—was very evident. On his left shoulder, two spots had bled and stained his pajamas.

Noting the irregular white scars that confirmed the chronic nature of this rash, I felt a growing sense of relief. Although a scaly rash on a geriatric patient can have many tricky causes, here, at least, there were no signs of skin cancer or secondary infection.

"You have neurodermatitis!" I bellowed.

Ralph nodded, his retriever barked an affirmation, and Mrs. Lewis arched her eyebrows.

I then explained that neurodermatitis occurs when skin becomes itchy from various causes, such as dryness or allergy. Repeated scratching leads to hypersensitivity and to a vicious "itch-scratch" cycle. Recommending the continuation of moisturizing creams, I said that I would prescribe hydroxyzine tablets to reduce Ralph's itching.

"Does that medicine come as a shot?" Mrs. Lewis was charitable but firm as she reminded me of Dr. Rucker's orthodox remedy.

I explained that hydroxyzine could be injected but that the pill form worked just as well. Writing out the prescription, I handed it to a hesitant Mrs. Lewis. "If the rash isn't better in a week, we'll try something else."

"That's fair enough, Dr. Jenkins. I'll be sure to let you know."

After bawling out our farewell to Mr. Tayson, his sister and I walked out of the room.

"You know, I think that Ralph's rash gets worse when he feels nervous," she observed. "He hardly ever gets out of this house. Without his dog, I don't know what he would do."

I nodded, thinking about the dozens of Ralph's kindred that I had seen before—sad, silent, and shrunken men slouched in wheelchairs and dozing in front of babbling televisions. In their colorless oblivion, they were living ghosts.

"It's good that your brother can be here at home," I said, "but I know it's a lot of extra work for you."

Mrs. Lewis's gray eyes penetrated mine. Lifting her chin, she seemed more erect than ever, and her pearls shifted slightly. "As long as I'm able, Ralph has a home. And," she added as if to squelch any doubts that I might have on the subject, "I plan to be able for a long time."

Following my hostess back through the solarium, I found myself in a spotless kitchen where Mrs. Lewis stopped abruptly. "Now before you leave, Dr. Jenkins, I want you to sit down and try my apple crisp."

Before I could answer, she opened her oven door and lifted out a casserole dish filled with simmering apples and topped with an oatmeal crust. The tantalizing aroma of apples, cinnamon, nutmeg, and brown sugar swirled around me in the room. My stomach issued a delighted growl.

"Oh, Mrs. Lewis! I should be going, but that does look absolutely delicious!" Pulling my chair up to the table, I glanced uncasily at the darkened windowpanes. Before I could speculate on whether the raindrops were turning to ice, I found myself sitting opposite Mrs. Lewis, separated only by two large china dessert bowls filled with steaming apple crisp. A pitcher of fresh cream materialized beside the apple crisp, and two cups of hot tea promptly followed.

Mrs. Lewis talked, laughed, and ate apple crisp. She recalled her days as an army nurse in World War II, her subsequent career as a high school biology teacher, and her retirement with her husband to Hebron Hill. When I complimented her roses and orchids, gray eyes sparkled.

"Have another helping of apple crisp," Mrs. Lewis urged with a knowing smile. "I was certain that you would like this dessert, Dr. Jenkins. I bought these apples from your mother just yesterday, and she always says that Stayman apples make the best apple crisp."

"I can't imagine how you could improve your recipe," I said guilelessly, watching her fill my bowl with a generous second serving.

Pouring on more cream, Mrs. Lewis talked about my mother and her apple orchard and about their long-standing commercial and social relationship. Then she talked about Madison County with its peaceful pace and idyllic mountain scenery. Between mouthfuls of apple crisp, I assented to her accolades.

Over an hour and a half after my arrival and completely stuffed with apple crisp, I donned my parka, and Mrs. Lewis opened the door. "This rain is turning to sleet," she remarked.

Stepping out onto the walk, I felt the treachery of a thin glaze of ice. "I probably should have left earlier. Your driveway is rather steep."

"Oh, but I'm so glad that you stayed! I don't think you'll have any trouble on my hill. Why, Dr. Rucker never did, and she's been up and down that driveway in all kinds of weather!"

Waving good-bye, I started down a driveway that was as slick as polished glass. Descending the slope in low gear, I knew that if I even grazed the brake, I would arrive at the bottom of Hebron Hill in an unprofessional tangle of truck, boxwood, and bittersweet. What would the effusive Mrs. Lewis say then about the new doctor who, during his first house call, had demolished her hedge and mailbox?

In my premonition, I listened as she relayed her story first to her homeowner's insurance agent, then to my mother, and then to all her neighbors. Slowly and cautiously like a novice skier making that petrifying first run, I crept down the hill.

Easing past the mailbox, I took a triumphant breath and congratulated my truck. "Good job, old fella! But just remember, if Dr. Rucker's Jeep could do it, so can you!"

CHAPTER THREE

MY MOTHER'S CRYSTAL BALL

No matter how old a mother is she watches her middle-aged children for signs of improvement.
—Florida Scott-Maxwell, *The Measure of My Days*, 1968

Three days later, on a crisp clear Sunday afternoon, I found myself driving alone toward the mountain farm that had been my boyhood home. My wife, Doreen, and I had returned from church with our four children only to have the telephone interrupt our Sunday dinner. A three-year-old patient was crying with an earache.

As I shoveled down the last few bites of lasagna, my family looked at me from around our kitchen table. After twelve years of medical marriage, Doreen had considerable tolerance for the quirks in my schedule, but since our move to Madison, the pattern of around-the-clock emergency telephone calls was a growing nuisance. While still adjusting to a different house and a different school, my children seemed also to be accepting that their father might be snatched away at any time and on a moment's notice. Grabbing my coat, I promised to join them at my mother's farm as soon as I could.

At the office, my clinical encounter went smoothly. After a few drops of anesthetic ointment in my young patient's ear canal and a prescription for an antibiotic, she skipped out into the November sunshine as if nothing had even been wrong. Her bleary-eyed parents thanked me and then headed home for a well-deserved nap.

As they walked toward their car, I glanced at my watch. The office visit had taken less time than I had predicted, and I celebrated my good luck. I would have enough time to drive up to the farm on the back roads.

As I guided my truck along the winding county road that obediently follows all the curves in the Robinson River, it felt good to be back home. Flanking the river on my left were long groves of sycamore trees, whose white trunks and auburn leaves swayed gently in the autumn breeze. On my right, the houses and barns looked very much the same as they had thirty years before when I was a first grader on our school bus.

In those simpler times, Madison County had been, for the most part, a network of small farms that were tended by the latest descendants of long-established families. But with the increasing tourism brought on by the national park, the price of adjacent farmland at first doubled, and then tripled, and finally increased by a factor of ten. As suburban government workers built their vacation cabins in what had for centuries been hayfields and orchards, they transmuted the rustic charm that they had grown to admire.

Almost all the farms are gone now. I reflected as I caught the first glimpse of my mother's apple orchard. Since my father's death several years before, my mother continued to operate the orchard that had once belonged both to her parents and to her grandparents. Never comfortable with her emotionally distant husband, my mother hardly seemed to notice that after forty years of marriage, he was no longer there.

But stubborn as she was, she was bucking the trend. All her closest neighbors were already gone. Lamenting the exodus of the farmers, a local newspaper editorial had commented that "the second Yankee invasion of Madison is worse than the first." My mother, glad to see her own sentiments in print, had taped this bit of parochial nostalgia onto her refrigerator door.

And there's Mom now, I thought, glimpsing a familiar figure standing by her garden gate. Parking my truck between two recently harvested apple trees, I walked over to join the stocky woman who was inspecting her prized perennial border. Even in mid-November, its hardy clumps of yellow chrysanthemums and purple asters offered a cheerful welcome.

"Well, it's about time you were arriving, Harold," my mother began as she leaned over to decapitate a dried aster flower. "Doreen and the children got here over an hour ago. They've gone for a walk up in the woods."

Crushing faded flower petals between callused fingers, my mother glanced at me and waited for my explanation. She had always believed in coupling her love with a substantial helping of severity.

"I had to run out to the office after lunch to check a patient." I tried to recreate the balance of apology and self-justification that I knew from years of experience was the best way to deal with my mother. "It was a little girl, Mom. She didn't sleep last night because of a bad earache."

Maternal lines softened as my listener looked down at the chrysanthemums. Golden in the late autumn sun, they were a tribute to her unrelenting attacks on the stony soil.

"Well, I suppose some people do need to see you on Sunday now and again." Mom was reluctant to allow the responsibilities of a medical practice to provide an excuse for her son's tardiness.

Reflecting on the clandestine pleasures of my ride by the river, I nodded.

"Doreen's already put a new electric cord on my iron," Mom continued. "The old one snapped last week, and she got it fixed in no time. And before she leaves this afternoon, she's going to adjust the front-end loader on the tractor. How your wife finds the time to raise four children and still take care of all the mechanical problems around here I'll never know."

Reflecting on my wife's reputation as Mrs. Fix-it, I shared Mom's sense of wonder. Before Doreen entered nursing school, she had been an assistant to her plumber-electrician father, and she continued to enjoy repairing appliances and machinery. My mother, who shared the meager mechanical aptitude of the rest of our clan, regarded Doreen as a technological wizard.

"And from what I hear about you," Mom continued, "you've been getting busier with every passing day."

"I've been working right along," I agreed, thinking back over the accelerating pace of my first month as a hometown doctor.

Almost from the beginning, my new medical practice had been a nonstop operation. In just a few weeks, Doreen and I had purchased a small office and begun a remodeling process that still was grinding along. The zoning administrator, high-handed in his petty bailiwick, had made us dig up the entire septic field; the highway department had forced us into a $50,000 bank loan to construct a paved turning lane; and the health insurance companies had buried us in paperwork. Somehow we had survived the onslaught and in a streak of beginner's luck had hired Ellen, who was an exceptionally quick and competent nurse.

Looking at my mother, I thought about the patient appointment sheets that were getting more crowded by the day. "Dr. Rucker certainly took care of a lot of people in Madison, didn't she?" I mused. "I had no idea that she had so many patients."

"Alma Rucker was completely overworked for her entire life." This assessment, coming from a farmer who toiled from sunup to sundown, was my mother's ultimate compliment.

But Dr. Rucker had lived in a different era, I brooded. Covering the entire county in her khaki-colored Jeep, she had delivered babies at home, saved life after life with antibiotic injections, and like a tireless professional relative had stayed up all night to care for and comfort the dying. To her many followers, she certainly had been somewhat more than human—and quite possibly only a little less than divine.

But from the safety of his tenured ivory tower in the medical school, Professor Matheson had declared that Dr. Rucker and her kind were the last of the Titans and that rural family medicine was a laughably impractical notion. Thinking now about the stack of bills growing ever higher on my office desk, I decided grimly that probably he had been right. What malicious star had led me, a generally cautious individual, to defy his wisdom in order to be a humiliating failure in front of my mother, my wife, and my huge extended family?

"I don't think you have a thing to worry about," remarked my mother.

I looked up so quickly that my neck snapped. From my earliest childhood, Mom's intuition had never failed to petrify me.

"With what everybody's been telling me," Mom went on, "I think you're getting off to a great start."

"You do?" I echoed, still coping with the uncomfortable sensation that my psychic mother could read me like a book. In the chemistry of the solid woman standing beside me was not one atom of either dishonesty or self-pity. Without fail, she spoke her mind, and her private doubts—if she ever had any—were off-limits even to her family.

My mother nodded. "Catherine Lewis called me again just yesterday. She's coming up tomorrow to get some more apples, and she told me that you'd been out to check on her brother. Catherine's always worshipped Dr. Rucker, but to hear her talk now, it sounds like you're going to work out just fine for her and Mr. Tayson."

I smiled as I pictured that diminutive but imperious lady and her china bowls filled with apple crisp.

"And in my opinion," my mother added with growing authority, "when either you or I can satisfy Catherine Lewis, we can probably satisfy almost anybody. Right now, she's singing your praises almost as much as she goes on about their new minister. Catherine thinks that Reverend Detamore can walk on water. But that's how the Baptists always are. For the first six months, their ministers can't do anything wrong, and then after that, they can't do anything right."

Bending over her flowers, Mom unwrapped the tendrils of a ground ivy plant that was climbing up an aster stalk and, with one determined movement, jerked the unlucky invader out of the ground and tossed it over the fence into the apple orchard.

"Well," I said, still trying to process my mother's unexpectedly rosy analysis of my professional prospects, "I think I'll venture out to the woods and link up with Doreen and the kids. It's a nice afternoon for a hike."

"Now don't you be gone too long." My mother relapsed into her familiar fusion of affection and reprimand. "I'm counting on a little time to see my grandchildren this afternoon. I don't get to be with my family as much as I'd like to anymore, and besides, Doreen will need some time to fix my front-end loader."

"I won't be gone long," I promised as I turned away from the garden gate to walk between rows of ancient apple trees that my great-grandfather had planted just after the Civil War.

Above me, on one carefully pruned bough, was a flash of color. Jumping as high as I could, I snatched from its twig a shiny red apple that the harvesters had missed. After polishing it with my handkerchief, I took a bite. Flavored by the frost, it was crisp, juicy, and delicious.

"Now this new medical practice," I said to myself as I munched on my apple, *"now **this** project is going to be real experience."*

"You mean it's going to be a real disaster, don't you?" In the jeering chorus of voices somewhere inside my head, I could identify Professor Matheson.

"Oh, it's going to work out fine!" retorted another inner voice that sounded suspiciously like my mother. *"Just wait and see!"*

Preoccupied by this internal duel, I strolled through the orchard until I reached a rusted wire fence. Across the pasture field—less than a hundred yards in front of me—rose the green and yellow wall of a poplar slope. From childhood, it had been my favorite retreat.

Cupping my hands to my face, I shouted into the silence of the familiar woods. "Doreen! Where are you?"

My echo bounced back just before my wife's reply. From somewhere above me on the mountainside came a muted response. "Up here!" Standing motionless, I heard in the distance the excited chatter of our children.

"I'm coming!" I yelled.

Clearing the barbed wire with a single leap, I suddenly realized that at least for now, my inner quarrel was over. As on so many other occasions, my mother had once again tackled the opposition and emerged the winner.

On this cloudless afternoon, it felt good to be back on the ancestral farm and to be breathing mountain air. Being a hometown doctor was going to be the hardest job that I had ever tackled, but now I was ready to hit it with everything that I had.

With lighter heart and quicker steps, I ran up the slope toward the oncoming sounds of laughing voices.

CHAPTER FOUR

THE SKETCH IN THE CHESTNUT FRAME

> **A man should keep for himself a little back shop, all his own, quite unadulterated, in which he establishes his true freedom and chief place of seclusion and solitude.**
> —Montaigne, *Essays*, 1580

It was Thanksgiving Day, but sitting alone in my medical office, I felt distinctly unthankful. On this holiday morning, I was previewing charts that were already pulled for Friday appointments. One chart belonged to Paul Crandall. With gloomy finality, I knew that its owner would not be coming in tomorrow.

During Paul's first visit four weeks before, Ellen, my homegrown nurse who prided herself on knowing all the interesting details about every Madisonian, for once was not a wealth of information. She did tell me that our new patient owned a vacation A-frame in Berry Hollow, adjoining the wooded slopes of the Shenandoah National Park. Her nursing note documented that he was fifty-two years old, unmarried, and having problems with his feet.

"Bunions, probably," Ellen advised. As she handed me the new chart, she polished her diamond and sapphire engagement ring. "After all, he's the right age."

Paul Crandall's pleasant crisp accent suggested New England. Dressed in tan corduroy trousers and a pinstripe oxford shirt, he was of medium build, and with his firm and ruddy face, he looked healthy. As he talked, he gestured with strong hands and asked me to call him Paul.

"I haven't seen a doctor for three years," my patient began, noting that at that particular checkup, an urban internist had pronounced his health to be excellent. Armed with this benediction, Paul had kept his distance from medical facilities. For the past twenty-one years, he had worked as an associate curator of an art museum. A few years ago, he had purchased his local vacation home where, when he was not tending his expanding plot of rhododendrons, he liked to sit on his deck and sketch the surrounding Blue Ridge Mountains.

"And that's what I would rather be doing today!" he commented wryly. "But I'm concerned about my feet and thought I'd better see you."

Paul then explained that about six weeks ago, he first had noticed some numbness in both feet. Initially, there was only a pins-and-needles feeling in both big toes. Thinking that his hiking boots were too tight, he had switched to a larger pair. Unfortunately, the discomfort had persisted and now was also becoming noticeable over his arches.

"Have you felt well otherwise?" I asked.

Paul assured me that, in a lifetime of good health, he had never felt better. He took no prescription medications, enjoyed a single glass of red wine before dinner, and walked on a regular basis. His favorite hike was the White Oak Canyon.

I chuckled. Located on National Park land in Madison County, the White Oak Canyon is a spectacular eight-mile stretch of clear mountain streams cascading over granite ledges. Surrounded by clusters of mountain laurel and flame azalea, it was one of my favorite hiking trails too.

On examination, Mr. Crandall appeared both younger and healthier than most men of his age. The only positive findings involved his toes, where he could not feel the light touch of a cotton swab. His sense of kinesthesis was also impaired. When I moved his toes up and down, Mr. Crandall couldn't describe the position changes unless he actually saw them. His muscle strength was entirely normal.

"You have the clinical findings of a peripheral neuropathy," I said. In this disorder, nerves for various reasons become irritated or inflamed and don't function properly.

"So what causes a neuropathy?"

Dipping deeply into the orthodox menu of causes, I served up a generous sample—diabetes, heavy metal poisoning, alcohol abuse, vitamin deficiencies, leprosy, and certain types of cancer.

Cautioning Paul that there were many other less common causes, I explained that the most important first step was to pinpoint a probable cause by checking a battery of blood tests and arranging an appointment with Dr. Dillon. This Charlottesville neurologist would perform a nerve conduction test, an electrophysiologic diagnostic procedure that identifies which nerve fibers are not functioning properly.

Throughout my lengthy medical monologue, Paul listened with interest. Readily agreeing to the blood tests, he deferred the neurology visit.

"After all," he reasoned with another wry smile, "I don't want to slide into the habit of visiting you doctors one after another."

"That's fine. I can call you with your results later this week."

"Oh, but I don't have a telephone." His calm eyes twinkled. "When I'm in Madison, I just want peace and quiet. How about if I come to the office to get my results?"

We shook on it, and my patient drove back to the red-and-gold glory of an October in Berry Hollow.

Paul's lab panel was completely normal.

"So that's good news, isn't it?" he commented as we talked together three days later.

Being an experienced medical pilgrim, I took refuge in professional ambiguity. "It is, and it isn't. Certainly, normal lab results are always reassuring, but without an explanation for your neuropathy, we won't be able to treat it effectively."

With a nod, Paul acquiesced. He would go see the neurologist.

"By the way, Doctor, I've done some reading since I saw you on Monday." At the University of Virginia Library, Paul had not been particularly pleased with his research. "There may not be any good treatment for neuropathy, isn't that right?"

Acknowledging that this was sometimes true, I noted that in almost every case, treatment was at least somewhat helpful.

"But if there is a really serious underlying problem, it may not be treatable. On Monday, you did mention cancer as one possible cause."

The blue eyes looking at me were grave, intelligent, and devoid of alarm.

"I also mentioned leprosy," I countered, "and I don't think you're likely to have either problem."

Paul laughed. "I do want you to know one more thing, Dr. Jenkins. I don't believe that a patient with a disease like cancer should have to agree to a lot of treatment that isn't likely to help. I remember my father's death."

His face told me that the memories were still very much alive.

"Dad was a smoker and had lung cancer. After the radiation and chemotherapy, he was completely miserable. He lost his hair, he vomited all the time, and after a while, I think that he was just hoping he would die."

I thought about my own father's lingering death from prostate cancer and about his oncologist's unflagging optimism, which at first had been heartening but eventually had become infuriating. "That must have been a very hard time for you."

Paul nodded. "And when I saw what Dad went through, I decided right then that I was never going to do that to myself."

I assured him that there was no reason to think that he was in a similar predicament. A consultation with Dr. Dillon would probably clarify the picture.

"Well, as a hiker, I do need to take good care of my feet."

"Perhaps that should be our therapeutic goal," I said with a laugh, "to keep you walking White Oak Canyon. After Dr. Dillon's consultation, I want you to come back to the office, and then we'll see where we are."

Agreeing with my plan, Paul then smiled shyly as he picked up a package that lay beside his chair. The size of a shirt box, it was wrapped in brown paper. "This is a little something for your new office, Dr. Jenkins. I thought that you might like a gift from Berry Hollow."

Peeling off the tape, I opened the box. "Paul, this is beautiful!" I exclaimed. In my hands was a framed black-and-white pencil drawing of a Madison County mountain landscape.

Pride glowed on my patient's face. "That's Buzzard's Knob, of course. I can see that ridge from my deck. And the frame is made from a native chestnut that had fallen in my own woods."

"This is the first piece of artwork in my office," I said. "Every time I see it, I'll think of hiking."

Two weeks later, I was finishing a well-baby check when Ellen knocked on the door. "Dr. Dillon's on line 1. I left Mr. Crandall's chart on your desk."

Right from his first word, Dr. Dillon sounded ominous. Agreeing with my diagnosis, he worried that this neuropathy was progressing more rapidly than usual. The nerve conduction tests showed a mixed sensorimotor pattern. Even though our patient was now feeling only numbness, his walking could rapidly become impaired.

"And I did send one more lab test," Dr. Dillon added. "This is an unusual neuropathy, Harold, so I sent an HIV titer. I'll let you know the result in a few days."

Hanging up the phone, I was stunned. In 1985, AIDS and other HIV-related diseases were certainly commonplace in American cities, but not in my isolated hometown. Jotting a few lines in Paul's chart, I went back to the cooing four-month-old. Although I returned her bubbly smiles, inside, I wasn't smiling.

Dr. Dillon's formal report arrived on the Monday before Thanksgiving. Sitting alone in my cubbyhole at the end of the workday, I read through three pages of technical language that confirmed our previous conversation. And under his signature, Dr. Dillon had scrawled, "HIV-positive. I've written the patient and sent him a return appointment."

In disbelief, I stared at the postscript. All around me, the darkened office held the hush of new fallen snow—or of a funeral parlor.

Closing my eyes, I said aloud the phrase that in 1985 was tantamount to a death sentence—"HIV-positive."

Glancing up at the chestnut-framed sketch, my mind was filled with thoughts of the artist. How would he handle this? How should I help?

In Berry Hollow, there was no telephone, and on that Monday evening, I considered this technical barrier with decidedly mixed feelings. On one level, I knew that I should talk to a patient whose life probably had disintegrated as he read his afternoon mail. But in a more cowardly way, I felt profound relief. I could not call Paul Crandall even if I knew what to say.

So sliding his chart into the outbox, I decided that I had three days to prepare for his upcoming appointment. Tomorrow, I would start by calling the University of Virginia Infectious Disease Service.

On Tuesday, I saw twenty-one patients before noon and was glad for a few minutes to gulp down my peanut butter and jelly sandwich. When the intercom buzzed, it was Ellen. "Dr. Jenkins, I'm sorry to interrupt your lunch, but the coroner is on the line. I'll bring you the chart."

In a few seconds, I was opening Paul Crandall's folder.

Without warning, the sandwich stuck in my throat as if some evil alchemist had changed it into a wad of newspaper. It was almost impossible to speak to Dr. Samuels, who, fortunately, was accustomed to doing most of the talking. Sipping on my iced tea, I tried to breathe and to choke down my lunch.

Dr. Samuels said that Mr. Crandall had died at home at approximately three o'clock this morning. A neighbor, Mrs. Hazelton, had stopped by the A-frame around ten o'clock to take Mr. Crandall along to a rhododendron society meeting. When no one responded to her persistent knocking, Mrs. Hazelton had opened the unlocked front door and had discovered the body. On the bedside table were two empty bottles—an eight-ounce container of chemical powder and a large bottle of Bacardi rum.

"Mrs. Hazelton says that they spray their rhododendrons with copper sulfate," remarked Dr. Samuels. "They call it bluestone and use it for a fungicide. I don't know what it does to the fungi, but it certainly does a number on people."

The coroner paused before adding. "Mrs. Hazelton says that Crandall had seen you lately for some type of podiatry problem. I don't suppose that you know why he might have wanted to commit suicide?"

****

Now, two days later, I sat in my abandoned lab and brooded over the finality of my clinical defeat. Ever since the coroner's call, I had been tormented by a question that never left me alone: *"Doctor, how could you have let this happen?"*

Through two sleepless nights, I had not devised a satisfactory answer.

Walking restlessly away from the counter, I looked again at the picture in the chestnut frame. Each careful pencil stroke recorded the characteristic features of Buzzard's Knob. On the north slope, a faint line intersected the trees. It was the hiking trail that Paul Crandall and I each had climbed on happier days.

"Maybe next time, I will do better," I pleaded with my merciless questioner.

"Maybe next time, Doctor" came the taunting echo from the wasteland of my guilt. *"Maybe next time."*

Suddenly, the picture entered the dialogue. In its detail, something new was standing out like a flashing neon sign. Moving closer, I examined my discovery.

In an accurate series of switchbacks, Paul Crandall's hiking trail wound around Buzzard's Knob, but as it crossed the bottom right corner of the drawing, it pointed to a message that I had missed before. Hidden among a thicket of oak trees was a diminutive but legible annunciation. "To Dr. Jenkins—Best wishes from Paul Crandall. November 3, 1985."

Suspended between gratitude and disbelief, I stared at the inscription. About Paul, there were many things that I didn't understand, but maybe, as a patient, he had been satisfied with my care. Maybe in his private world, he had never wanted me to be Superman—the hero who would crash into his life with redemptive force. Maybe he had simply lived and died in the way he wanted to. And maybe that was okay.

Finishing up the chart reviews, I walked out to my truck. In the west, the rugged cliffs of Buzzard's Knob stretched up toward a clear November sky. On this morning, so saturated with life and death, I felt thankful again—thankful to be close to the mountains and to be heading home for Thanksgiving.

CHAPTER FIVE

CORONARY ANGIOPLASTY AND BARLEY GREEN TEA

It is always the best policy to speak the truth—unless, of course, you are an exceptionally good liar.
—Jerome K. Jerome, *Idler Magazine*, February 1892

"What you need is fenugreek tea. That's the best thing for a sore throat."

At her checkout counter, Mrs. Eula Umstadler was speaking in earnest. "Now if you develop a cough along with your sore throat, it's better to mix horehound with the fenugreek. It works faster."

The customer, nodding her appreciation, paid for the chicken salad sandwich and the two packages of recommended herbs.

"And I know you'll feel better soon," said Mrs. Umstadler approvingly. "My herbs are so much better than prescription medications."

As I sat at the oilcloth-covered table and munched my pork barbecue, I knew that Miz Eula was pleased that I patronized the restaurant that she operated along with her husband, Wade.

At Umstadler's, the homemade food was unfailingly excellent. Wade's sister, Olive, got up at three o'clock every morning to mix, knead, and bake all the breads. Olive also created the desserts that were displayed on glass shelves under the counter—fresh apple pies with sugar-glazed crusts, deep-dish blackberry cobblers, and lemon pies piled high with meringue from the Umstadlers' own homegrown eggs.

Wade, an easygoing six-footer, flipped steaks on the grill and also operated the ever-busy deep fat fryer. Topped by a thatch of graying hair and in his early fifties, he looked older because of the forty extra pounds around his middle. An occupational hazard, I decided. If I cooked at Umstadler's, I would probably have to be weighed on a truck scale.

Miz Eula, however, was undeniably different. Surrounded by her spare-tire husband, her pleasantly plump sister-in-law, and her overweight clientele, Mrs. Umstadler stood out as a model of dietary self-control.

Although pictures of multiple grandchildren smiled down from the knotty pine paneling, Miz Eula herself did not look matronly. She sewed her own size 5 dresses, which always had modest sleeves and low hemlines. Her wavy silver hair, parted uncompromisingly in the middle, crowned a placid face whose lips were somewhat thin.

A single-minded businesswoman, Miz Eula relegated all public relations duties to her good-natured husband. While Wade found it easy to banter with his customers, Miz Eula was more comfortable when she was near her cash register with its large adjoining rack of herbal remedies.

Basic to Miz Eula's personal raison d'être was her belief in the healing power of herbs. Years ago, she had accepted her duty to minister to her ailing fellow citizens, and she had carried out her mission well.

At the first sign of cough, rash, or constipation, local sufferers promptly consulted Miz Eula, who, with the accumulated wisdom of her years, dispensed herbs and advice. After her customers purchased packages of dried tansy, chamomile, and feverfew, they would often sit down in the restaurant to take their first doses along with steaming bowls of homemade chicken noodle soup. Leaving an hour later, they were often amazed to realize how much better they already felt.

Of course, in the unlikely event that their symptoms should linger, they could always squander hard-earned cash and go see the local doctor.

Day after day, as I savored my hot lunches, I became increasingly aware that Miz Eula relished her role as my health-care competitor. Soft-spoken by nature, she tended to project her voice toward the local doctor's table.

"For restoring circulation, there's nothing that can beat rose hips," she declared to the elderly couple who were paying their restaurant bill. "And elderflower tea will prevent colds. It's better than a flu shot." Placing her remedies in a brown paper lunch bag, she congratulated the couple and then shot me a look of quasi-religious triumph—alternative health care had once again beaten the Big Brother.

As a lifelong gardener, I actually shared some of Miz Eula's enthusiasm for herbal treatments, but obviously, for her, the boundaries were clear. She had already drawn her line in the sand. And although I was a regular at their restaurant, the Umstadlers never returned the favor. Probably as owners of a booming business, they didn't have time to come to my office. And given the spectrum of Miz Eula's expertise, few medical problems could be beyond her reach.

For constipation, Miz Eula dispensed crushed flaxseed, and for diarrhea, a formulation of powdered angelica root. She attacked the gray specter of depression with lavender flower tea and dried vervain; she banished insomnia with regular doses of valerian; and she tamed unruly menstrual periods with evening primrose oil. She could even stimulate a flagging appetite with a blend of ginseng and apple mint tea.

And although Miz Eula did not stock any weight reduction aids, I attributed this omission not to a gap in her professional ability but rather to her prudence as a restaurant owner.

So on that busy Friday afternoon, I was genuinely surprised when Ellen handed me a thin new chart. "Wade Umstadler is here with chest pain. I'll get an EKG."

The EKG was fine, and at 146/80, Wade's blood pressure was normal. He was on no medications.

I sauntered into the exam room. "Hello, Wade! It's nice of you to finally visit me!"

At the end of his long day, Wade looked a little tired but was still good-natured. "It's probably nothing, Doctor, but I didn't feel exactly right this afternoon, and I thought I'd like to see you before I went home."

Shortly after his usual large lunch (today's special—Olive's meatloaf along with lima beans, mashed potatoes, and gravy), Wade had felt some tightness in the center of his chest. On other occasions, he had experienced indigestion, but this afternoon, four Mylanta tablets hadn't helped.

After lunch, he had unloaded a delivery truck and had carried heavy cases of canned food up the back stairway. "That's when it really got bad. When I was going up those steps, I felt so much chest pressure that I had to stop and sit down. And then after a while, it started letting up, and finally, it went away completely."

"How long did you feel the chest tightness?"

Wade pursed his lips. "The worst of it was about fifteen minutes, but I guess it lasted over an hour."

I asked if the chest discomfort had seemed to travel toward his arms or neck.

"Never into my arms," he replied, "but when it was at its worst, I felt an ache in my left jaw. That's when I felt really bad—weak, sweaty—like I might black out."

As I examined Wade, we kept talking. No, he had never had any previous episodes of chest pain and, in fact, was rarely ill. His parents had died of old age, and the only heart attack in the family had nailed an elderly uncle who was an incorrigible cigarette smoker. Wade himself had never smoked. He also had never had high blood pressure or diabetes.

I slipped my stethoscope back into my lab coat pocket. "Your physical exam is okay, and your EKG is normal."

My patient's face brightened.

"But you still need to be admitted to the hospital, Wade. You may be having a heart attack."

"But I feel fine now," my patient objected. "The pressure is completely gone."

"I understand, but you still belong in the hospital." I then explained to him that his symptoms of chest tightness, jaw pain, weakness, and sweating were very suggestive of angina, the type of chest pain caused by a blockage in normal coronary blood flow.

"With the right treatment in a coronary care unit," I persisted, "we can sometimes prevent a heart attack."

Wade studied the brown carpet. "Okay," he said finally. "You're the doctor."

Our office moved quickly. Ellen called the Rescue Squad—the dispatcher promised that a volunteer team would be at our office in twenty minutes—and then placed an oxygen cannula on her patient's nose.

On the telephone, I reviewed Wade's situation with the University of Virginia's on-call cardiologist, Matt Eisenberg. As medical students, Matt and I had spent four hectic years together. This afternoon, he would be waiting for my patient in the CCU.

"It's all set up for you, Wade," I announced. "The Rescue Squad will be here soon. So now you probably want to let your wife know what's going on."

Simple Gifts

As I handed him the extension phone, my patient hesitated. "How about if you call Eula, Doc? You'll be able to explain everything so much better than I can."

Although it was already a few minutes past the restaurant's closing time, Miz Eula answered after only one ring.

"I'm glad that we caught you before you left, Mrs. Umstadler," I began. "I need to tell you that the Rescue Squad will be taking Wade to the hospital. He seems okay right now, but I'm concerned that he may be having a heart attack."

Miz Eula gasped and then was silent. Buttressing my explanation with details, I reviewed my office evaluation, complimented the Rescue Squad, praised Dr. Eisenberg, and then paused to accept her concurrence.

"I don't see any reason for Wade to go to the hospital," her dry voice responded. "He's probably just having another attack of indigestion. Wade never told me that he was going to your office. I thought he was at the bank. If I had known, I would have fixed him up myself with some catnip tea."

Like a bad attack of vertigo, the exam room whirled around me. Perhaps I hadn't made myself clear. "Mrs. Umstadler, I'm here with your husband now, and I don't think his problem is indigestion."

"Well, you said yourself that his EKG was normal." Miz Eula's voice was chilly. "And besides, there's never any reason to go to a hospital on a Friday afternoon. They won't do anything for you over the weekend. If you think Wade needs a heart test, he can have one on Monday."

Reeling under this barrage of objections, I looked over at Wade. With his eyes closed, he was taking deep breaths of oxygen and maintaining a diplomatic detachment from my telephone skirmish.

Now, of course, I understood why Wade had wanted me to tackle Miz Eula. During my years of emergency medicine, I had frequently informed wives about their husbands' heart attacks. Until this moment, I thought that I had already experienced all possible spousal reactions—shock, grief, anger, panic, incredulity. But never before had I encountered the disdain that I was getting from Miz Eula.

"Doctor, we don't have health insurance," she said accusingly. "Medical care costs so much that average working people just can't afford it."

With a cough, I acknowledged my own culpability, and she went on. She still saw no reason for Wade to go to the hospital. She was sorry that he had bothered me.

Now that I understood why she was reluctant to send her husband to the hospital, I had to act fast. Groping around for options, I suddenly realized that my alternative health-care antagonist had dealt me a playing card.

"Mrs. Umstadler, I think that I understand where you're coming from. The county depends on your restaurant, and you have to keep it open." As a generally honest physician, this was my all-time champion whopper, but somehow the situation begged for a harmless lie.

I then suggested that since Dr. Eisenberg was already available to see Wade, it might save the Umstadlers time to go to the hospital now. That way, they wouldn't have to be away from their restaurant next week.

I had plunked my trump card onto the table. Now I waited. On a professional level, I was glad that Mark Eisenberg hadn't overheard my sales pitch that was as flimsy as it was deceitful.

"Well, okay, Doctor." Mrs. Umstadler was begrudging. "We'll do it your way. Tell Wade that I'll go on home to do the chores and then pick him up at the hospital this evening."

"I'll be glad to." I was elated to hear the sharp metallic click as she hung up.

Right on cue, Wade opened his eyes. "Is Eula all right?"

"She's fine. She's going home now, and she'll meet you at the hospital."

Ten minutes later, Paramedic Rob Thorson had packed our patient securely into his ambulance and with a wave of his giant hand had headed down the highway. It had taken a lie to do it, but I had won my card game with Miz Eula.

On the following Monday morning, our office was the usual zoo. Both the parking lot and the exam rooms were packed, Ellen and I shot past each other in the hall, and the telephone rang incessantly. Dr. Eisenberg's call made it through at eleven o'clock.

As always, Matt was affable and complimentary. Praising my decision to send Wade to the CCU, he chose not to add that only a brain-dead physician would have done anything else.

Shortly after arriving, Wade had experienced recurrent chest tightness. An emergency cardiac catheterization had revealed a nearly complete thrombosis of the left anterior descending coronary artery. After emergency angioplasty, Wade had done well with no further chest pain and with his enzyme tests revealing no evidence of heart damage.

"So I'm discharging him this afternoon," Matt concluded. "He's to cut his weight, take an aspirin every day, and see you in a week. I'm certainly glad that he came in when he did."

"That makes two of us," I agreed.

That week, the office was so busy that I didn't get away for lunch until Wednesday. As I stepped out into the cold November air, it felt good to be facing another homemade meal at Umstadler's.

From behind the grill, Wade spotted me immediately. "I feel great today, Doc!" He grinned.

Several lunchtime customers stopped eating long enough to wave to me. From her station at the cash register, Miz Eula managed what could have been a weak smile. Obviously, for her, this was an awkward moment.

But the food was as grand as ever. Blessed with the Southern mountaineer's hearty appetite, I waded into the steaming split pea with ham soup, complete with a plate of hot buttered rolls. As I devoured my lunch, several customers paused at the cash register, accepted their herbal packets from Miz Eula, and walked out into a world of guaranteed well-being.

Finally, after savoring the last crumbs of Olive's blackberry cobbler, I walked over to the counter where Wade was standing beside his wife. "I really appreciate everything you did for me, Doc," he said softly. "It feels good to have you here so nearby just in case I ever need you again."

"But, of course, you're not going to have any more trouble," Miz Eula said, correcting him. "I've put you on a diet. Cottage cheese and peach slices today, wasn't it?"

Tallying my bill, she refocused her attention. "And besides, Doctor, I'm giving Wade barley green tea three times a day and a fresh grated ginger root at bedtime. He should be fine, don't you think?"

Before I could answer, I looked past Miz Eula to catch a glimpse of Wade's face. Many times before, I had witnessed his trademark grin, but this was the first time that I had ever seen his wink.

I felt both complimented and astounded.

"Oh, I do think you're probably right, Mrs. Umstadler," I said with what I hoped was a proper degree of professional deference. "And thanks for another wonderful lunch. I'll see you again soon."

CHAPTER SIX

ON SEDATIVES AND CHURCH ATTENDANCE

> **For it is with the mysteries of our religion as with wholesome pills for the sick, which swallowed whole have the virtue to cure, but chewed, are for the most part cast up again without effect.**
>
> —Thomas Hobbes, *Leviathan*, 1651

"Needs medication refilled." This brief chart note offered Ellen's entire explanation for the initial office visit of Mrs. Alice Stover, the next patient on my afternoon appointment sheet. The chart also told me that Mrs. Stover was sixty-two, married, and the operator of a dairy farm.

"Hello, Dr. Jenkins. It's nice to meet you." A tanned robust woman offered a warm handshake. With sensible brown eyes, rosy cheeks, and friendly wrinkles, she looked like a farmwoman. Her bobbed hair—sandy and flecked with gray—looked like it spent a good deal of time under a baseball cap.

After our introductions, Mrs. Stover proved to be a flowing conversationalist. Soon I had heard about her husband, her two grown daughters, and her grandchildren. Her only previous surgery, a hysterectomy, led to annual gynecology follow-ups.

"I must be in great shape!" my patient reported with a laugh. "I help milk seventy cows twice every day, and I drive our tractor more than I do my car. Really, I just never have any medical problems."

"But you do need to have a medication renewed?"

"Yes, I do, Dr. Jenkins." My patient lowered her voice. "Before she retired, Dr. Rucker always wrote my prescription, and she warned me to never run out of Valium."

Instantly, I was fascinated. Mrs. Stover just didn't seem to be the type of person who regularly would use tranquilizers. Her eyes intercepted my surprise.

"Oh, I don't use Valium very often, just on Sunday mornings." For at least ten years, Mrs. Stover had taken a five-milligram tablet about an hour before leaving for church. Somewhat sheepishly, she noted that she never needed this medicine at any other time.

In fact, when she arose on the typical Sunday, she felt fine. After milking the cows, she cooked sausage and hotcakes, tidied up the kitchen, and then started to dress for church.

And that was when my patient usually noticed a dry mouth and a vague sense of uneasiness. If she shamed herself into not taking the Valium, she would make it to her pew where she would feel flushed, dizzy, and nauseated. Sometimes her heart fluttered, and she wondered if she was going to die right there in church.

No, she never blacked out. She never had similar symptoms at other times, such as during dental treatments. She had never described her symptoms to anyone except her husband and Dr. Rucker. Of course, rich in native common sense, she had never seen a counselor and wasn't planning to start now.

We talked for a few more minutes, and then I wrote an order for fifty Valium tablets. As Mrs. Stover tucked the prescription into her bulging leather satchel, she told me that she would be back to see me in another year. With a wave, I hurried off down the hall.

Two weeks later, a local celebrity arrived for his initial office visit. When I spotted the Reverend Mark Detamore's name on the appointment book, I thought about my mother's comments about the popular new minister of the Deep Run Baptist Church. Ellen was eager to prime me with a spate of additional information.

Reverend Detamore was thirty-eight years old and had played football during his college years in Alabama. Engaging, handsome, and with a likable family, he had swept his new parishioners right off their feet. After years in the doldrums, Deep Run Baptist Church was now packed every Sunday. And today the man behind the miracle was coming in to have a prescription filled.

"How are you, Reverend Detamore?" I welcomed the strapping six-footer with his firm handshake and clear blue eyes.

"Glad to meet you, Doctor," the newcomer drawled. "I'm doing fine. Just call me Mark."

After an enjoyable chat about our backgrounds and our families, I turned to the business at hand. "And so you need a prescription refilled?"

Reverend Detamore's broad face colored. "Yeah, phenobarbital. I take a tablet every Sunday morning before I preach." Digging into his pants pocket, he produced a well-worn medicine bottle.

"How long have you been taking phenobarbital?"

Clearing his throat, Mark told me that he had first used this medicine because of stage fright in seminary. And even now, after fifteen years in different pulpits, his voice still tightened when he looked out at an audience.

When I confessed my own wariness of public speaking, Mark grinned as if we had shared a boyhood secret. He took no medicines other than phenobarbital. His regimen called for one tablet before each Sunday service, one and a half tablets before a funeral, and two tablets before a wedding. Laughing at his gradation of various occupational stressors, I refilled his prescription.

Broad shoulders bowed in appreciation, and as I watched them disappear down the hall, I knew that I had just encountered an unusually dynamic man. No wonder that the Deep Run folks were so elated. Thinking about the introverted monotone who read his political polemics from our Methodist pulpit, I sighed.

Just five days later, our church choir arrived as guest musicians at the Deep Run Baptist revival. In the rural South, the annual revival is as legendary as fried chicken, and we arrived early to allow adequate time for the superb potluck supper. Mark Detamore slapped me on the shoulder before introducing me as "my new doctor friend" to the guest evangelist, Brother Clifton. This luminary was considerably older and more somber than Mark, and they seemed to be a little uneasy with each other. But all three of us had excellent appetites, and we enjoyed overeating together.

Our choir settled into the platform chairs ten minutes before start-up time and watched the church fill up with people. Deep Run Baptist Church, constructed before the Civil War, is trimmed in native walnut that gleamed in the light from the antique chandeliers. On the top of the spinet piano was a porcelain vase of winter greenery. Suddenly, there was a tap on my shoulder.

"Why, hello, Dr. Jenkins!" It was the friendly face of Alice Stover, welcoming both me and the choir before she sat near the front of the sanctuary.

Even after collective gluttony, our choir sang with gusto. As we launched into "Beulah Land," congregational feet were tapping on the old pine floor. By the time we belted out the final refrain of "Just a Little Talk with Jesus," the Deep Run folks were whistling and clapping. This was their type of music!

But now the merrymaking was over, and it was time for that formidable centerpiece of every revival, the evening sermon. After Brother Clifton's five-minute opening volley, I knew that we were in for it.

The evangelist depicted himself as God's chosen messenger, and the message was clear—God was annoyed with contemporary society in general and with the Deep Run folks in particular.

I listened only halfheartedly to Brother Clifton's barrage of sadomasochism. Like most other Southerners, I had heard all this before. As emotions go, guilt is not particularly long-lived.

But the evening dragged on, and the captive audience stared into their laps at hymnals, church bulletins, and funeral home fans. On the front pew, three sullen teenage boys chewed gum and shuffled their tennis shoes. In the velvet-trimmed pulpit chair, Mark Detamore's sprawling athletic frame was relaxed. With brimstone raining down around him, he was at peace with the world.

Directly in front of me, three rows back in the congregation, was Alice Stover. Casually wafting away Brother Clifton's apocalyptic warnings with her fan, she looked untroubled—even serene.

"And why shouldn't they both feel good?" asked an impertinent little voice inside my head. "You would be relaxed too if you had taken a Valium or a phenobarbital before you came here this evening."

Even for a Methodist intruder at a Baptist revival, the little voice was inappropriate, but he was so much more entertaining than the sermon that I gave him my full attention.

As a physician, I had prescribed for both Mrs. Stover and Reverend Detamore sedatives for them to take specifically before they came to

Simple Gifts

church. Of course, before this evening, I hadn't realized that they both attended the same church, but here we all three were at a revival, and I was the only one that was feeling uptight.

Trapped in my pew, I listened to the seductive little voice. "Really, Doctor, is churchgoing such a stressful activity that it requires premedication like outpatient surgery? Maybe you religious people should station a parish nurse in the narthex just to administer your anesthetics!"

Somewhat reluctantly, I conceded that the little voice had raised a legitimate point. Had I really been correct in prescribing sedatives for either Alice or Mark?

Perhaps when we come to church, we shouldn't have to wear masks—even pharmaceutical masks. Maybe a church needs to be nonthreatening, the ultimate sanctuary where we can risk being transparent and real.

My flight of fancy vanished with Brother Clifton's abrupt shift of intonation. "Now turn in your hymnals to Number 402. Let's sing all five verses of 'I Surrender All.'"

With voices appropriately solemn and subdued, we pledged ourselves to forsake all earthly pleasures and to pursue a number of other equally unlikely projects. After a closing round of pulpit formalities, I escaped with my choir folder into the delightful fresh air of the churchyard.

But driving homeward in my truck, I was still thinking about Mrs. Stover and Reverend Detamore.

Due to a vicious attack of poison ivy, Mrs. Stover actually didn't achieve her promised full year's absence from my medical office. Only a few weeks after the revival, she had weeded her periwinkle border and was now covered with contact dermatitis.

"Doctor, we certainly enjoyed having your choir sing at our church." My patient's cheerful facial symmetry was somewhat distorted by large red whelps. "Why, I had no idea that my doctor could sing!"

That physicians are untrainable in all fields except medicine is such an embedded cultural conviction that I try never to directly address it. Instead, I perjured myself by commenting that I had enjoyed my recent evening at Deep Run.

Alice Stover was more honest. "Actually, it was just awful. You can only imagine how much I dread our revival. It's the only week in the year that I use a Valium every day."

Secure in my diagnosis of poison ivy, I didn't feel rushed. "Have you ever thought about telling your minister that you take Valium before you go to church?"

Mrs. Stover looked both startled and amused. "Oh, Reverend Detamore would never understand how I feel! He's such a wonderful man, always calm and matter-of-fact. Why, he never feels nervous about anything! I'd be too embarrassed to admit to him that I do."

I pushed on past her eulogy. "Sometimes all of us feel that way about being up-front with our ministers, but maybe we shouldn't. Maybe it would be better for everybody if we just said what we really feel."

My Baptist patient looked skeptically me. After all, I was a Methodist. "I don't know, Doctor. I can't even think of a reason to tell Reverend Detamore why I would need to talk to him."

"Why not just tell him that your new doctor advised it?"

Suppressing a smile, I looked down at her chart. "And now let's talk about your poison ivy!"

CHAPTER SEVEN

THE OCTOPUS'S ASTHMA ATTACK

> The family—that dear octopus from whose tentacles we never quite escape.
>
> Dodie Smith, Dear Octopus, 1938

"We have a new asthma patient coming in," Ellen said as she added another entry to the appointment sheet. "Arlene Butler."

"Why, I know her," I said, recognizing the name of one of my younger cousins. By now, Arlene was probably twenty-five, but she was still plagued by the allergies that had appeared in her early childhood. Usually, she went to a pulmonary specialist in Charlottesville.

After only a few minutes, Ellen's urgent summons interrupted my dictation. "Dr. J., I need you right now."

"Coming!" Shoving back my desk chair, I bounded through the cubicle door.

Just outside the exam room, Ellen looked worried. "Arlene's having a really bad asthma attack. I've already started two liters of oxygen, and as soon as you check her, I'll give her a nebulizer treatment. I sent her mother out to the waiting room."

On the exam table, a slim brunette—sitting bolt upright—was breathing rapidly. To hear her wheezes, I didn't need my stethoscope.

I chucked the usual Southern social niceties. "How long have you been sick, Arlene?"

"For two weeks—I started an antibiotic—last Thursday—it isn't helping. I'm a lot tighter today." My patient's history came in staccato phrases interrupted by gasps. I grabbed my stethoscope.

"Take deep breaths with your mouth open," I said. My stereotyped instruction was complete nonsense. Arlene's mouth was already wide open, and her chest and neck muscles were fully mobilized.

Over my patient's right lung, I heard loud wheezes—the high-pitched whistling of the bronchospasm that was part of Arlene's asthma. Over her left lung, I was surprised to hear no wheezes. In fact, I heard nothing at all.

"We'll give you a nebulizer treatment right away." I checked my cousin's medication bottles—an inhaler, an antibiotic, and some bronchodilator tablets. "Have you been taking your medicines regularly, Arlene?"

From behind the vapor-filled face mask, my patient nodded. Consumed with the work of breathing, she wasted no energy on talking.

"Dr. J., her axillary temperature is 103," Ellen reported. "Arlene, have you ever had pneumonia before?"

Our patient shook her head. "No—never pneumonia—just bronchitis."

Ellen adjusted the oxygen mask. "Is your nebulizer treatment helping?"

"A little—I think."

"The next thing we'll get is a chest X-ray," I announced. "Arlene, I think you have pneumonia. You're going to need to go the hospital. I'll talk with your mother."

Walking slowly toward the waiting room, I thought about the inherent awkwardness of being a physician for one's own relatives. Given the vast size of my extended family and the shortage of local physicians, I often treated relatives for their minor sprains and sore throats. Today marked my first encounter with a life-threatening situation.

Since my childhood, Arlene's mother had been my Aunt Lillian—the sturdy countrywoman whose identity was wrapped up in the bleached tea towels waving on her clothesline and in her neat rows of red and white petunias.

For the weddings, funerals, and other major events in her extended family, Aunt Lillian's contribution was always the same—a moist yellow pound cake baked with a dozen brown eggs, flavored with lemon extract, and drizzled with sugar glaze. No sorrow was too sudden, and no celebration too elaborate, to be met without one of Aunt Lillian's pound cakes.

And now I was facing my first adult conversation with a person who had always related to me as her younger brother's second son—one more member of our extended clan. I glanced out the lab window at the white pines in our office yard. In the afternoon breeze, they swayed like graceful ballerinas.

Squaring my shoulders, I marched into the waiting room. "Aunt Lillian, I need to talk to you about Arlene. Let's walk back to the hall."

The familiar maternal figure in the pink floral dress and the home-knitted white sweater stood promptly. Replacing the issue of *Southern Living* in the magazine rack, she picked up her oversized purse and walked in front of me at her usual deliberate pace.

On our way down the hall, I signaled to Ellen. "Call the Rescue Squad. Tell them to come stat."

Aunt Lillian looked puzzled. "Harold, do you really think that Arlene needs to go the hospital? She's had asthma all her life, but she's never had to be admitted for it before."

Wham! My evolving treatment plan had just suffered a head-on collision with frank skepticism. My aunt was a force to be reckoned with.

"Aunt Lillian, I know that you've had a lot of experience with asthma, but this is not just an asthma attack. I think that Arlene probably has pneumonia too."

"Well, she has been sick all week," my aunt conceded. "Finally, this afternoon, she let me bring her to the doctor."

When she pronounced the word "doctor," Aunt Lillian looked hesitant, almost embarrassed as if she might have chosen the wrong title. When her gaze shifted from my nametag to my face, I could only imagine the intellectual somersaults that were going on inside her head. I watched as she walked back to the waiting room.

The nebulizer treatment didn't help Arlene. When I stepped back into the exam room, my cousin was breathing more rapidly than ever, and her face was tight and anxious. Ellen slipped the X-ray onto the view box. "This X-ray looks odd to me. What's wrong with it?"

Although technically a good film, it indeed was an odd X-ray. Where my patient's left lung should have been, there was only a white blur. We were looking not at the air that was usually there but at the fluid that had displaced it.

And there was another odd thing—the configuration of the chest was all wrong. My cousin's heart and major blood vessels had shifted noticeably away from the midline toward her right side. The fluid around her left lung was interfering with her circulation and was putting dangerous pressure on her right lung, where all the work of ventilation was now occurring. In its black-and-white silence, Arlene's X-ray screamed at me from the view box. "Life-threatening, life-threatening!"

Instantly, I snapped out an order. "Get the crash cart!"

In a flash, Ellen darted through the door to return with the tray that contained all our equipment for major emergencies.

"Arlene," I said, looking directly at my cousin, "I need to put a needle into your chest. You have a lot of fluid around your left lung, and it has to be treated now. It can't wait until you get to the hospital."

Fighting for breath, Arlene nodded. The desperation in her feverish eyes was a blend of hope and doubt—mostly doubt.

"Give me 5 cc of Xylocaine with epinephrine," I ordered. Ellen handed me the medicine. "Arlene, you're going to feel a stick."

As I injected the medication subcutaneously, the white wheal of anesthetic spread out from my needle. Repositioning the syringe just below the margin of the left second rib, I injected Xylocaine through the chest wall, through all three layers of intercostal muscles.

"Betadine and four by fours," I ordered.

Ellen handed them to me. With ever-widening strokes, I scrubbed my patient's chest with the brown stain of Betadine antiseptic.

"Get a basin ready," I said.

Ellen grabbed a blue plastic one from the nearby shelf. With one rapid movement, I pushed my large-bore needle deeper and deeper into Arlene's chest wall. Suddenly, I felt a reassuring pop. I had penetrated the pleural cavity.

Gripping the hub of the pink plastic catheter, I pulled out the metal needle. From the catheter shot a whoosh of pressurized air, followed by a thin stream of foul yellow fluid that hit the basin with enough force to make me jump.

"It's empyema fluid," I commented. The thick exudate, with its mustard yellow color and putrid odor, was spurting rhythmically into the basin after each of my cousin's exhalations.

"You should be breathing better soon," I said to my patient. "The Rescue Squad will be here in a few minutes."

In the venerable annals of medical communication, my telephone conversation with the University of Virginia Emergency Department stands out as a model of brevity. A twenty-four-year-old asthmatic patient with pneumonia had presented to our office in extreme respiratory difficulty.

I had decompressed her tension pneumothorax, and a large amount of empyema fluid was currently shooting from her chest catheter.

"Arlene will be flying to Charlottesville," I told Aunt Lillian. The University emergency department was dispatching the hospital's medevac helicopter, *Pegasus*. "And she's going to be okay. In fact, she's a lot better already."

And by the time that Rob Thorson bolted into the exam room, Arlene was comfortable enough to offer the giant paramedic a weak smile.

"What on earth is this thing, Doc?" Rob pointed to my patient's chest catheter. Draining more slowly now, thick yellow fluid oozed from the plastic opening.

"Don't worry about what it is," I snapped. When a doctor has just saved the life of one of his relatives, he doesn't need to take the time to educate a paramedic.

Rob looked appropriately subdued.

The ambulance transfer from our office to the helipad went smoothly. Alerted to the family crisis, my mother was waiting for Aunt Lillian at the high school parking lot that doubled as the county's helipad. Five minutes later, *Pegasus* and Arlene had lifted off for Charlottesville.

As the helicopter disappeared above the treetops, Aunt Lillian turned toward Ellen and squeezed her hand. "I can't tell you how much I appreciate everything. I knew that Arlene was sick, but I never realized just how very ill she was."

Ellen patted Aunt Lillian's forearm. "She's going to be okay. I'm so glad you brought her in when you did."

"You did exactly the right thing, Lillian," my mother agreed.

When my aunt stepped toward me, her rubber-soled shoes squeaked on the pavement. But for that background noise, I might have heard the scraping of her mental gears. "Doctor Jenkins, how can I thank you enough for everything? It's so good to have you here in Madison."

As I processed the new level of respect in Aunt Lillian's voice and looked at the pride in my mother's eyes, I felt good—very good.

"And, Harold," my aunt continued, "I'll be by the first thing tomorrow morning to drop you off a pound cake."

My mouth watered in anticipation of another warm-from-the-oven treasure. "Now you don't have to go to all that trouble, Aunt Lillian."

"It's no trouble at all," declared my aunt as she tossed her handbag onto the rear seat of my mother's car. "I'm always glad to bake a pound cake for a special occasion. And if this isn't a special day, what is? You're my nephew, you're Arlene's doctor, and you deserve it."

As Mom and Aunt Lillian drove away, Ellen winked. "And so, dear Doctor, I'll be skipping my shredded wheat tomorrow morning. You are going to be sharing that pound cake with me!"

CHAPTER EIGHT

MRS. MARSHALL'S SURPRISE

> To live in this world
> you must be able
> to do three things:
> to love what is mortal; to hold it
> against your bones knowing
> your own life depends on it; and when the time comes to
> let it go,
> to let it go.
> —Mary Oliver, "In Blackwater Woods"

As I drove down the winding country road, Christmas lights twinkled from trees, shrubs, and doorways. In the twilight, hundreds of ornaments—red, green, and blue—painted their patterns on the snow like watercolors running together on a palette. On one festive lawn, electric bulbs outlined an oversized doghouse that was crowned with a flashing star.

Until now, today had been exceptionally enjoyable. At lunchtime, I had played my first tennis match with Mark Detamore, the new Baptist minister. Only last week, Mark had suggested a get-together, and I had jumped at the chance.

Returning to the office after our game, I felt exhilarated by the physical workout and by the range of my new friend's intellectual interests. Here, for the first time since my return to Madison, was the promise of camaraderie.

But now the fun was over, and I was on my way to Mountain View Nursing Home to meet my first resident patient, Mrs. Mamie Marshall.

Driving slowly over the icy patches that dotted the roadway, I thought about the long-gone nursing home patients of my medical residency. Most of these elderly people had been severely demented, and our initial encounters were usually frustrating monologues. I remembered an assortment of age-stricken faces—confused, apathetic, tearful, and often bewildered.

And I suppose that Mrs. Marshall will be much the same, I mused as I parked my truck. *After all, she is ninety-two years old.*

Treading cautiously over the frozen parking lot, I walked through a door decorated with magnolia and holly branches. The hothouse atmosphere of the lobby and the odor of Lysol stirred up unpleasant memories.

After ringing the bell at the vacant front desk, I glanced at a display cabinet filled with rag dolls, embroidered snowflakes, and colorful potholders. A modest sign, hand printed in all capital letters, told me that the residents sold these craft items to raise money for their picnics and shopping trips. Thinking back to residency days, I couldn't recall any nursing home outings.

From around the corner came the hurrying footsteps of a friendly young nurse. Wearing a pristine uniform and a Mennonite prayer cap, she smiled her welcome. "You're here to see Mrs. Marshall, Doctor?"

I nodded.

"I think that she's really going to enjoy living here. She does such a lot of needlework. I helped organize her quilting supplies this afternoon."

My face betrayed my surprise. "I didn't realize that Mrs. Marshall was so active. She is ninety-two, isn't she?"

Commenting that my newest patient wasn't one to act her age, the nurse led me down a paneled corridor decorated with Impressionist landscape paintings. Under our feet, the polished tile floor gleamed like a black-and-white checkerboard. Stopping outside a closed oak door, my companion tapped softly.

"Come on in," a sturdy voice invited.

Walking over to the tall big-boned occupant of the wheelchair, the nurse introduced me as the new physician, patted Mrs. Marshall's shoulder, and left the room.

"Why, it's so nice to meet you, Doctor." My patient's Southern Appalachian drawl was untarnished by the standard diction of nationwide

Simple Gifts

TV shows. When she smiled, dozens of tiny wrinkles animated her broad face. Above gold-rimmed spectacles, her ivory hair was thick and wavy.

"Haven't had many dealings with doctors myself," said Mrs. Marshall with good-natured tolerance. "In my time, I've had fourteen children, and I delivered every one of them at home. Why, after each one came, I just cut the cord with my sewing scissors. Why would anyone bother to have a doctor do that?"

"Is this your family picture, Mrs. Marshall?" From a brass-framed photograph, four long rows of faces smiled out at me.

"Sure is," my patient affirmed with a contented chuckle. "Have you ever seen such a crowd? That was my ninetieth birthday party, and there I am, right smack in the middle of it."

I looked again at the photograph. Sure enough, Mrs. Marshall—embellished with a pink-and-white carnation corsage—was beaming back at me from the front row. "You certainly have a nice-looking family."

Mrs. Marshall assured me that she was proud of all of them. Her first ten children had been born in Marshall Hollow before the family homestead had been annexed into the newly formed Shenandoah National Park. After the Marshalls' eviction, four more children had arrived, followed by a small army of grandchildren, great-grandchildren, and great-great-grandchildren.

"Mrs. Marshall, how do you ever remember all their names?"

With a laugh, my patient told me that she never forgot a name. Still, should she ever need a memory aid, she kept one nearby. Pointing to a shelf, she asked me to hand her the largest of several quilts.

As I helped unfold her handiwork, it covered the entire bed and spilled over onto the floor. In finely stitched triangles, a sturdy family tree stretched exuberantly across a sunflower yellow background. On a multitude of twigs was the roster of Mrs. Marshall's descendants.

"Why, this is a masterpiece!" I declared. "It must have taken you forever to finish it."

"Oh, only two months. Usually, I can finish a quilt in one month, but the embroidery on this one took a little longer."

In response to my query about her current project, Mrs. Marshall showed me a blue and gold wedding ring quilt. Her favorite pattern, it was to be a wedding gift for Ruth Ann, one of her great-granddaughters. With a gnarled index finger, my patient located Ruth Ann's perch on the family tree.

"With so much energy, you must have always enjoyed good health," I commented. My patient noted that arthritis, which had first started to bother her at age seventy-five, had been, in fact, her only serious problem.

Troubled by increasing pain, she had undergone several joint replacement surgeries. Six months ago, while pouring water into a birdbath, she had slipped and broken her left hip. After that operation, she had never been able to get around without her wheelchair. Since two of her friends were already Mountain View residents, she had decided to join them.

When I helped my patient onto her bed, she placed two pillows under her knees and one behind her neck. Covering her cream-colored nightgown were long rows of embroidered teddy bears—each one holding paws and smiling broadly.

Other than her advanced destructive arthritis, Mrs. Marshall's physical examination was surprisingly normal. But while her blood pressure, heart, and lungs were unremarkable, even a slight movement of her left hip caused a grimace.

"Well, you've already found the spot, Doctor!" As she congratulated me, her wrinkles brightened. "I feel so lucky that the arthritis isn't in my hands. I can still do needlework all day long."

My patient took only one medication—a daily pill for her arthritis. Agreeing to continue that medicine, I suggested that she try as much as possible to stay physically active in the nursing home. Mrs. Marshall gave me a kind but superior look.

"I've been active all my life, Doctor, and I certainly don't intend to change anything now. When you've raised fourteen children, you don't have time to be lazy."

The four faces of my own energetic offspring flashed in front of me. Jotting a note on my new patient's chart, I suddenly felt a deep respect for this woman's success. Certainly, I could not imagine the destabilizing impact of ten more children on our already-bustling home.

When I conceded that Mrs. Marshall never could have been lazy, she hastened to provide supporting evidence. When she and her husband were married in 1908, she was sixteen, and her husband was eighteen. Together, they had sawed down the trees that provided the beams and boards for their house and barn. Mrs. Marshall herself had split the chestnut logs that became the rail corrals for their hogs and cows. Her garden—over an acre of potatoes, corn, beans, greens, and squash—had fed her family throughout the year.

As her string of children grew ever longer, she incorporated their care into the daily rhythms of her farmwork. The boys had climbed the Blackheart cherry trees to shake the sweet fruits onto bedsheets spread out on the ground below. The girls had sorted out the twigs and leaves, and Mamie had sold dried cherries by the pound at the local store. In the fall, she sold chestnuts and dried apples, and year-round, she marketed eggs, cream, and homemade butter.

I studied the family tree quilt. "It must have been very hard for you when the Park took your farm."

When Mrs. Marshall responded, her voice was calm and even. Indeed, it had been more than hard. After losing a homestead that had been in his family for generations, her husband had never gotten over his bitterness. Although the Marshalls had moved only a few miles away, he never went back to see what the Park had done to his hollow. Twelve years after the eviction, he died in defeat, a prematurely old man.

"Have you ever been back to the farm yourself, Mrs. Marshall?"

My patient indicated that she had returned only once. The summer after her husband's death, she had developed an irresistible urge to see everything just one more time.

"And how was it?"

"Oh, nothing like it had been, that's for sure. The Park had burned our house and all the outbuildings, you know, and almost all the fences were gone. I did find our spring. That water was always as cold as ice, and it never slowed down even in the worst dry weather. Down below it, there was always a good patch of watercress, and when I went back, there they were, still growing away. Some of the apple trees had a little fruit on them, but that was years ago. I expect everything is gone by this time."

I thought about the nostalgia of a neglected apple tree—an eloquent statement of some farmer's lost dream. "And so you've never been back to your hollow since that one visit?"

Mrs. Marshall shook her head. "Always been too busy doing something else, Doctor. I'm not one for dwelling in the past. The present is plenty good enough for me."

My patient eyed me through gold-rimmed spectacles. "I'll just tell you what I've always told my own kids. When we have something, we need to enjoy it like a gift—to hold it and touch it every day. But when it changes, we need to go ahead and let it go. Something else will come along before long."

Looking at my patient's gentle wrinkles, I thought about how much she had enjoyed and how much she had let go. "I think you're going to do quite well here, Mrs. Marshall. I'll be back next month to check you again."

"Well, I'll be looking forward to seeing you, Doctor." My patient rebuttoned her teddy bear nightgown, and I helped her back into the wheelchair. When I left, she was smoothing out the wrinkles in the family tree quilt.

As I checked the column of boxes on the admission form, the nurse walked over to the desk. "Doctor, isn't Mrs. Marshall remarkable for a ninety-two-year-old?"

"I expect that she was remarkable at any age."

Thinking about my patient's cascade of surprises—her good humor, her creativity, her optimism—I smiled at my own reply. Against all my expectations, I had enjoyed my evening at the nursing home and was looking forward to my next visit with the surprising Mrs. Marshall.

CHAPTER NINE

AN OFFICE CHRISTMAS EVE WITH JIMMY

> **A conscientious doctor must die with his patient if they can't get well together. The captain of a ship goes down with his ship into the briny deep, he does not survive alone.**
> —Eugene Ionesco, *The Bald Soprano*

"Oh, holy night, the stars are brightly shining!" The lyrical soprano solo filled our sanctuary as I accompanied our choir on the organ. Softened by the glow of candlelight and by the nostalgic fragrance of cedar and bayberry, our colonial church on this Christmas Eve echoed the timeless benediction of peace on earth.

After the postlude, I walked over to accept the soloist's hug. Her eyes shone with the wonder of a starlit night in Bethlehem. My own eyes were bleary after an unexpectedly busy day.

"I enjoy Christmas music," I commented, "but it feels really good to have it over with. This week's been awfully hectic."

In fact, an epidemic of streptococcal sore throats had raced into Madison just in time to ambush the holidays. Our office had been so overrun that I had skipped dinner in my rush to get to church. Still ahead of me were three shiny new bicycles waiting to be assembled before I could go to bed.

Preoccupied by the thousands of nuts and bolts that are essential parts of three bicycles, I offered halfhearted greetings to my mother and

Aunt Lillian. Decked out in seasonal finery, neither one seemed to notice anything amiss.

As I hung up my choir robe, someone raced up the back steps.

"Oh, Dr. Jenkins, I'm so glad that you're still here!" Mary Mullins, an alto choir member, was out of breath. "My little Jimmy just fell in the parking lot. I think he needs stitches. Can you take a look at him?"

Mary's five-year-old son whimpered as he sat on a stool in our church kitchen. Carefully removing the white washcloth, I looked at the jagged two-inch laceration across Jimmy's left eyebrow.

"That will definitely need stitches," I agreed. "Who's your pediatrician?"

"Dr. Booker. But he's all the way in Charlottesville, and I really don't want to go up there on Christmas Eve." Mary eyed me hopefully. "Could you take care of Jimmy in your office?"

I thought about my postponed dinner, the unassembled bicycles, and the deeper meaning of the season.

"Sure," I replied. "It shouldn't take long to fix this little problem."

Walking back into the sanctuary, I discovered Doreen enjoying her favorite hobby. With her opened tool chest resting on the pulpit, she was repairing a microphone that had faded out during the church service. Always awed by Doreen's mechanical wizardry, Mom had agreed to drop our children off on her way home.

After promising to be home by 10:30 p.m., I drove down the snow-covered road toward our office. "This won't take very long," I said, comforting my rebellious stomach. "I really need to get home."

Inside the office door, Jimmy stalled.

"Let's go around to the exam room," I proposed.

Spurning my invitation, Jimmy grabbed his mother's legs and hung on. Mary—after begging, wheedling, and threatening her offspring—finally hauled him bodily into the exam room.

"This won't take long, Jimmy," I repeated as I arranged a surgical tray on the Mayo stand.

My patient looked doubtful, and on reexamination, I began to share his misgivings. The laceration was unexpectedly deep. At its base gleamed the shiny white surface of Jimmy's frontal bone. I would need to close the cut in layers.

At no time in a medical office is a nurse more essential than during a minor surgical procedure. As I filled the syringe with local anesthetic, I thought of Ellen, celebrating the evening with her family. While I soldiered on alone, my nurse probably was sitting by a cheerful fireplace; an overflowing bowl of hot popcorn would be nearby.

And here I was with Jimmy. From the depths of Mary's red and green Christmas dress, my patient stared out at me like a frightened bear cub.

"Now, Jimmy," I continued brightly, "I need to put some medicine in your cut so that it doesn't hurt anymore. Can you climb up here on the table by yourself?"

Not one to suffer fools gladly, my patient buried his tousled red hair in his mother's dress. After exchanging glances, Mary and I hoisted him onto the exam table. In thirty seconds that reverberated with Jimmy's objections, I anesthetized his laceration. The first phase of our tête-à-tête was over.

As I unfolded a blue surgical drape, Jimmy's whimpering abruptly stopped. "What's that?"

Explaining that the drape provides a clean work area, I asked Jimmy to lie down. With reluctance written all over his freckled face, my patient flattened out on his back. As a tactical strategy, Jimmy had chosen to cooperate as long as everything went well.

"Nothing's going to hurt you now," I assured him. But as I dipped some gauze pads in a basin of Betadine, I could tell that our détente was becoming shakier by the second. Assuring my patient that the brown antiseptic was painless, I swabbed the margins of his laceration.

As I picked up my irrigation syringe, I suddenly realized that I had forgotten to pour any saline into the basin. In my heart, I cursed my carelessness and thought of the ever-efficient Ellen.

Looking at Mary, I smiled. "I just need one more thing." Pulling off my sterile gloves, I retrieved the saline from the top shelf, regloved, and double-checked the tray. Everything was in order.

"Jimmy doesn't have any evidence of a skull fracture," I advised as I palpated his frontal bone. "I'll flush the area, and then we'll be ready for stitches."

From her chair, Mary smiled as she held her son's hand. Basking in her goodwill, I suddenly felt glad to be a good neighbor on Christmas Eve. *Peace on earth*, I thought. *This is what it's all about.*

Tearing open my suture packet, I stared in disbelief at its contents. The thread was not the familiar blue filament that I expected but rather a thick tan one. In my haste, I had grabbed the wrong type of suture. Several unseasonal expletives flitted through my head, jostling for space with my Noel sentiments.

"I need to get a different type of suture," I announced as I discarded a second pair of gloves and walked over to the supply cabinet. Across the miles, I thought I could smell Ellen's buttered popcorn. I regloved and tried again.

Jimmy tolerated my false starts with commendable composure. Without difficulty, I placed a row of sutures in the facial muscles and then started to pull the subcutaneous tissues together.

"You're doing great, Jimmy," I said, snipping the ends off my surgical knots. "We'll be done in just a few more minutes."

Through the oversized drape, Jimmy's left eye maintained its cyclopic vigilance. Over everything, Mary's smile was a gracious beatitude.

And then without warning, it happened—the disaster that destroyed my Christmas Eve. Eying Jimmy as I reached for a gauze pad, I felt my hand strike the edge of the Mayo stand. The top-heavy tray swayed, tottered, and then fell to the floor. The resounding crash rang in our ears.

Jimmy leaped to his feet, tore off the enveloping drape, and joined his mother and me in surveying the array of surgical supplies scattered over the exam room floor.

Noncommittally, I commented that I was glad that such mechanical failures were infrequent. Stepping around forceps, syringes, scissors, and clamps, I selected a dry path to the supply cabinet, pulled down a second tray, and added fresh supplies.

Only by intense diplomacy was Jimmy lured back onto the table. As I placed the needle in the holder, I worked deliberately, always apprehensive of what might go wrong next. Inside myself was the deepening conviction that my gesture of Christmas goodwill was evolving into a public relations disaster.

Under his spreading blue canopy, Jimmy looked like a camper in a backyard pup tent. Against my renewed promises of a swift conclusion to our rendezvous, his skepticism radiated out in palpable waves.

"You're being a really big boy," Mary said, patting her son's arm. "Santa will be proud of you."

Glancing down at the debris-covered floor, she added rather unconvincingly, "We'll be on our way home soon."

Sweat dripped from my hands as I picked up the forceps and the needle holder. Just now, these familiar tools of the trade seemed alien to me like I had never seen them before. Ever on guard against another clumsy mistake, I finally clipped the last suture.

"Jimmy, you have eighteen stitches." The relief in my voice was unprofessional. "Just stay right there until I get a bandage."

Stepping back from the Mayo stand, I pivoted on my heels and headed toward the cabinet. In a flash, I realized my mistake. I was seeking traction in a sticky pool of Betadine. Desperately, I tried to stop, but it was too late.

With arms flailing, I traversed the room in an impressive slide that terminated only when my right knee slammed into the cabinet. Sensory overload exploded. Simultaneously, I felt burning pain, heard cabinet shelves rattle, and saw two unopened surgical trays plunge to the floor. Sterilization tapes snapped, and the tray contents flew in all directions, tripling the mess on the exam room floor.

Not even these cataclysmic occurrences were enough to distract me from the main event. Crouching in orthopedic agony, I watched as little Jimmy launched himself from the exam table. With the drape flapping behind him like the leathery wings of an ancient pterodactyl, he flew into his mother's lap.

In their own way, my two companions offered a contemporary variation on the Nativity motif. But in my office, the serene infant of the medieval paintings was transformed into a young patient in full-blown panic. Even the Madonna looked a little ruffled.

"Are you okay, Dr. Jenkins?" Mary's tone was chilly.

"Oh, I'm fine!" Tentatively shifting my weight, I was relieved that my right knee held me up.

Taking infinite care, I circumnavigated the landlocked sea of Betadine, staying well away from the treacherous reefs of partially submerged medical instruments. Trying not to wince, I hobbled over to the mother and child and like a bedraggled Magus offered my bandage.

As I peeled off Jimmy's drape, he was fused to Mary. Without incident, I squirted a thin line of antibiotic ointment onto the laceration and covered it with the nonadhesive bandage.

"Your stitches will be ready to come out on Monday," I said.

The angle of my patient's chin made me glad that Ellen would be working that day. I would certainly need a lot of help to hold this bambino down.

The three of us made the pilgrimage to the front desk. I limped, Mary walked, and Jimmy rode on his mother's hip, clutching her purse like a soldier gripping a hand grenade.

"Two o'clock on Monday afternoon," I said, handing Mary an appointment card. Through flashes of pain, I kept my right leg ramrod straight and tried to be festive.

"Have a great Christmas, Mary!" I said. "Jimmy, see you on Monday!"

Through the holly-trimmed door, Mary and her boy-child vanished into the night. Standing in the freezing air, I listened to the crunch of shoes on packed snow and then to the rumble of a departing car.

Back in the lab, I dropped into a chair. With dull foreboding, I rolled up my soiled suit pants. If I needed stitches myself, I would have to drive to Charlottesville. I had already used up all my own surgical trays.

When I glimpsed the ugly bruise, I sighed with relief. I could put some ice on that at home. Unlocking the medicine cabinet, I downed two aspirin tablets. Then like a reveler who has enjoyed too much eggnog, I staggered back to the disaster area.

The exam room that had been immaculate only two hours ago now looked like an emergency department after a bus collides with a train. Opened surgical trays were everywhere, and medical instruments cluttered the floor. On the exam table lay a crumpled surgical drape that apparently had been marinated in Betadine.

Resting on my good knee, I gathered up all the loose instruments and then like a lame workhorse hauled them back to the lab sink. I wasn't looking forward to Ellen's court of inquiry on Friday morning, but for now, it was the best I could do.

Picking up a box of absorbent blue pads, I hopped back to the scene of my Christmas misadventure and began to clean up. After multiple basins of hot soapy water, I had restored the exam room to a reasonable image of its former self. From underneath the supply cabinet, some Betadine still taunted me, but with my lame leg, that mess would have to wait.

When I got home, I eased out of my truck and half-walked, half-crawled up the front steps. As I hobbled through the front door, my wife's cheerful voice floated out from the kitchen. "Welcome home! What took you so long?"

Forgoing a rational reply, I collapsed onto the recliner. "Bring me an ice pack. Make it a big one."

Running into the living room, Doreen stopped in front of my chair. With silent misgiving, she completed her inspection of me and my ruined suit pants.

Simple Gifts

"I'll get you an ice bag right away." She patted my blue knee. "And I bet you're going to be glad that I've already finished putting those bicycles together. You can stuff the stockings while you're icing your knee."

My wife stepped back from her wounded warrior. "And just one more thing," she said as she pointed toward the mantel clock. It was 12:01.

"Here's a kiss for you, dear," said Doreen with a smile. "Merry Christmas!"

CHAPTER TEN

A DIET PLAN FOR MRS. HOLMES

**It's a very odd thing—
As odd as it can be—
That whatever Miss T eats
Turns into Miss T.**

—Walter de la Mare, "Miss T.," 1913

"And now you're going to meet one of my relatives, Dr. J." As Ellen pointed to a brand new chart, she shot me a cryptic smile. "Aunt Harriet has decided that she needs to lose a little weight."

And don't we all, I thought as I remembered the cheeseballs, ham biscuits, and pound cakes of the recent holiday season. After multiple family gatherings, the church social, and a New Year's Eve party, I was definitely well nourished. Even my twice-a-week tennis duels with Mark Detamore had not been enough to preserve my usual contour. Pulling in my paunch, I walked into the exam room.

"Mrs. Holmes, it's nice to meet you."

Extending her hand, my patient tried to disengage her portly figure from the exam room armchair. As I watched the struggle, a mass of vertically striped navy blue polyester rotated and twisted on its axis like a determined protozoan oscillating on a microscope slide. After a series of shifts and turns, Mrs. Holmes lunged forward and was finally standing upright.

"I have always wanted to know why every doctor's office has such uncomfortable chairs," she said accusingly. "You all must get them from the same factory."

I chuckled as I gripped my patient's plump hand. From her head to her feet, Mrs. Holmes was a series of expansive curves and folds that would have been a challenge for any seat smaller than a sofa. Her face—pink and chubby—was supported by a neck that was as thick as it was long. Her arms were hefty, and her ankles spilled over the sides of her glistening black shoes. Even her fingers were endowed with natural padding. Each digit was a line of bulges that tapered out to a manicured crimson fingernail.

"I've decided to lose some weight," announced Mrs. Holmes as she eased back into the offending chair. "That's why I've come to see you today."

Looking at my patient's overflowing frame, I acknowledged that she had identified a reasonable goal.

"And that's where you doctors aren't very much help," declared Mrs. Holmes with a reproachful nod. "My problem is not my pituitary or my thyroid or one of those other glands. I've already had all of them checked any number of times. But I do think that my blood pressure would be lower if I dropped a few pounds."

"I'm sure you're right." To carry calories to all of Mrs. Holmes's far-flung cells, her arteries must be working overtime.

"In fact," my patient continued, "I'm beginning to lose patience with the entire medical profession. Why, I've been going to see doctors for years, and my weight stays exactly the same."

"So you've had a weight problem for a long time then?"

"I certainly have." Mrs. Holmes looked at me through long-suffering eyes. "Of course, I didn't have the problem when I was growing up. Back then, I was as skinny as the other kids."

As I looked at the distinct cupola of fat that crowned each eyelid, it was hard to imagine that Mrs. Holmes had ever been skinny.

"It all started when I got married," my patient continued, frowning at her wedding ring. "It's all Albert's fault when I think about it. Now if you men had to give birth to all the children, we women would be able to keep our figures."

I decided against apologizing for gender-specific biological prerogatives. God and Darwin would have to fend for themselves. "And has your weight stayed about the same over the past several years?"

"More or less." My patient sighed. "I usually stay right at 220."

Glancing down at Ellen's chart note, I eyed today's measurement—232. "And like most of us, you are a little heavier after the holidays."

"Doctor, I do not weigh 232 pounds! There's something badly wrong with your scales!"

While I commented vaguely about sensitivity variation in medical instruments, the figure in the armchair scowled. Possibly if in the seclusion of her own boudoir, Mrs. Holmes had laid aside her heavy-duty girdle and several yards of polyester, she might have trimmed the disputed measurement by a few pounds, but her massiveness would have still been undeniable.

"So how much do you say that I should weigh?" Her tone was unforgiving.

Clearing my throat, I referred to statistical tables of weight ranges based on height and gender.

"And, of course, the recommendations are higher for men and lower for women, aren't they, Doctor?"

Thinking once more of the enviable remoteness of God and Darwin, I agreed that they were. "How tall are you, Mrs. Holmes?"

"Five feet six inches," she retorted. In our hearts, we both knew that it wasn't enough. To accommodate her present bulk, Mrs. Holmes would need to be over nine feet tall.

"So for you," I said, eyeing my pocket-sized chart, "the recommendation is that you weigh between 135 and 150 pounds."

The armchair convulsed erratically. "Well, at least I was normal on my wedding day. Doctor, it just isn't fair. I'll never be able to lose that much weight."

Slipping the maligned document into my pocket, I suggested that perhaps if we used the chart only as a guideline, Mrs. Holmes still would be able to achieve a worthwhile weight reduction. This, in turn, would decrease her risk for multiple medical problems, including diabetes and heart disease.

"Of course, of course," Mrs. Holmes chided. "So here's my question. What are *you* intending to do to help me lose weight? You're my new doctor, and all the other ones have been no help at all." A curiously hybrid look of regret and self-satisfaction spread over her face. "No, no help at all."

"Well, I'll be glad to offer some suggestions."

"That will be fine, Doctor. I'll sit right here in this chair and listen to what you have to say." And with an expectant look, Mrs. Holmes folded her hands and closed her eyes.

At first, I thought she might be praying. Perhaps, given the failure of all earthly physicians, this wasn't such a bad idea. But as the seconds ticked by, my patient continued to look like a dreaming Buddha.

Realizing that I had missed an important cue, I scrambled into a homily about the medical and social spectrum of obesity. In describing weight gain as the inevitable result of an imbalance between calorie intake and energy expenditure, I noted that as most of us grow older, we tend to exert less and eat more. After embellishing my talk with statistics and anecdotes, I stopped and waited.

In the armchair, eyelids fluttered and then slowly opened. Mrs. Holmes looked like she was emerging from general anesthesia. "I've heard all that stuff a hundred times before, and none of it ever works. Dr. Jenkins, I hardly eat anything anymore, and I still can't lose an ounce. Why, this morning for breakfast, I had a cup of black coffee and half of a grapefruit."

Looking more and more like St. Catherine on the wheel, she added, "And for lunch, I had a cup of unflavored yogurt and the other half of the grapefruit. I tell you, Doctor, I can gain weight on fresh air and ice water."

Glancing at my watch, I decided not to be sidetracked by the marvels of Mrs. Holmes's metabolism. Certainly, for researchers into the problem of world hunger, her case report suggested a promising new angle, but that was for another day. "What exercise program have you tried?"

Mrs. Holmes's glance was withering. "Now as weak as I am from my daily diet, how am I supposed to *exercise*?" She pronounced the last word as if it were a gutter-level expletive. "I suppose that soon, you'll be telling me that I ought to run two miles every day."

Instead, I suggested a more moderate aerobic program while cautioning my patient to continue her dietary effort. "You'll need to keep in mind that when you walk two miles, you're only burning off the calories that are in two slices of bread."

"I don't eat two slices of bread in a week," Mrs. Holmes rejoined. "And I've forgotten what homemade rolls and butter even look like!"

Pushing doggedly along toward some elusive endpoint, I urged my patient to record her daily food intake during the next two weeks and then to come back so that we could review her progress.

"I'd rather try something else, Doctor," objected Mrs. Holmes. "Why can't you just prescribe a pill that will help me shed a lot of this weight?"

Why not, I thought. *Why are humans so willfully blind to the interface between self-discipline and good health? Why are we obsessed with losing weight as long as it involves no lifestyle changes?*

Fortunately, in January 1986, there were no widely accepted medications for weight reduction, and I explained this to Mrs. Holmes.

"Well, I'm not surprised," she said, shaking her head. "But while you doctors keep wasting so much research money on everything else, you'd think that someone would spend a few dollars to help people like me."

I stood up. "We'll talk more in two weeks."

Again, Mrs. Holmes tussled with the armchair and after some noteworthy gyrations emerged the winner. "I'll bring in that calorie count, Doctor, and then you'll see what I mean. I'm practically starving to death."

Escaping through the door, I reflected on my patient's parting warning. Somehow Mrs. Holmes's eminent demise from malnutrition seemed very improbable, but unfortunately, so did the likelihood of my therapeutic success. Obesity rivals alcoholism as a challenge to the family doctor.

Two days later, as I strolled into the lab with the last of the morning's charts, I suddenly realized that I was famished. "Let's run down to Umstadler's," I said, thinking happily about my favorite local restaurant.

In a few minutes, Ellen and I were sipping tall glasses of iced tea while we contemplated the arrival of two orders of the Friday lunch special—roast beef, mashed potatoes with gravy, buttered corn, and cheese squash casserole, accompanied by a plate of Olive Umstadler's hot homemade rolls.

"And I always enjoy the dessert that comes with the Friday special," I enthused. "Olive's chocolate cream pie!"

"You love all of Olive's desserts," Ellen said with a laugh. "But then from the size of the crowd in here today, you're not alone." Leaning out of our booth to view the multitude, she grabbed my arm. "Why, even Aunt Harriet is here today! There she is with a friend of hers, only two tables away. Let's go over and say hello."

Before I could reply, my nurse was out of her seat. Reluctantly, I trailed after her. I really wasn't looking forward to a lunchtime chat with Mrs. Holmes.

And obviously, Aunt Harriet had not been anticipating a surprise encounter with me. As we approached her table, I witnessed her startled reaction. Her plate was piled high with the Friday special, and she was holding a buttered roll in midair. When she spotted me, she looked guiltily at the roll, wavered for a moment, and then returned it to her bread plate.

"Why, Aunt Harriet!" Ellen cried. "It's so good to see you again. This makes twice in one week!"

Mrs. Holmes blushed as she explained that her friend had invited her out for lunch.

"The food here is wonderful, isn't it, Mrs. Holmes?" I said. And then with malice aforethought, I added, "I especially enjoy the homemade rolls!"

"Oh, Harriet really likes them too," her friend assured me. "She's already eaten three, and that's number four there on her bread plate."

Mrs. Holmes's face turned from pink to red to purple, her eyes widened, and her hands trembled. For one dreadful moment, I thought that she had aspirated and that I would be using my Heimlich maneuver right there in Umstadler's Restaurant. But Mrs. Holmes was not choking. In fact, both her color and respirations quickly normalized, but for some strange reason, she remained unable to talk.

"Well, you enjoy your lunch now!" Ellen said as she leaned over and kissed Aunt Harriet. "And say hi to Uncle Albert for me."

Back in the booth, our own lunch was excellent. Soon, Olive was bringing us two thick wedges of chocolate cream pie. Looking over her shoulder, she asked about the heavyset lady who had just vacated the other table.

"Oh, that's my Aunt Harriet," Ellen replied. "She lives over in Orange."

"Well, I don't mean to pry," Olive said, apologizing," but I just thought that she didn't look so very well when she left. She didn't finish her roast beef, and she never even touched her pie. Do you think she was feeling okay?"

Before Ellen could answer, I interrupted. "Oh, she'll be fine, Olive. She probably just ate more rolls than she should have."

I paused as I stuck my fork into two inches of chocolate cream pie. "But it really is too bad that she didn't eat her dessert. I know she would have enjoyed it!"

CHAPTER ELEVEN
THE CRAYON DRAWING

If there is anything that we wish to change in the child, we should first examine it and see whether it is not something that could better be changed in ourselves.
—Carl Jung, "Vom Werden der Personlichkeit," 1930

"Dr. J., I'm putting a lot of green ink on your afternoon schedule."

Ellen's bulletin had undertones of regret. Taped to my desktop was a tricolor appointment sheet—blue for scheduled appointments, red for emergency add-ons, and green for walk-ins. In our office, green was everyone's least favorite color.

"Actually, this walk-in is a family affair." Ellen explained that the Crummetts were new to our office. Two of the four children were waiting for me in the exam room.

I asked Ellen why she had brought them back from the waiting room before their charts were ready. This was an inefficient deviation from protocol.

"You'll know when you go in there." My nurse pinched her nose. "They're not the cleanest children I've ever seen, and I just had to get them out of the waiting room."

There is something unforgettably distinctive about the body odor of filthy people. As a farm boy, I grew up around cows and pigs, but no barnyard animal can match the pungency of the unwashed human. And at this moment, the exam room was bulging with unwashed humans—five of them.

"Hello, I'm Dr. Jenkins." I was an island of antisepsis in a sea of grime.

A tired-looking woman extended her hand. Although she was probably in her early twenties, her eyes were much too old for the rest of her face. Her figure—petite becoming pudgy—was not flattered by a dingy yellow dress. Her only adornment was a silver wedding band.

"I'm Mollie Crummett," she said rather uncertainly, "and these are my children." A row of thin bodies tapered across my exam table. Light green discharge was dripping from all of their noses, and their raspy coughs filled the air.

Since Mrs. Crummett didn't offer any further introductions, I asked which of her offspring were Iris and Loretta.

"That's them!" the oldest child declared. The stridor in her young voice was startling. "That's Iris and Loretta. They're twins!"

"Well, thank you! And what's your name?"

"I'm Dixie!" My informant wiped her nose on a frayed sleeve. "I'm the oldest, then there are the twins, and last of all is the baby. He's Cletus!"

Pulling out a tissue, I handed it to Dixie. "Can you tell me how old everyone is?"

Dixie blew her nose and then stuffed the crumpled tissue into her pocket. "I'm the oldest," she repeated. Pride of primogeniture glowed on her grubby features. "I'm six, and Iris and Loretta are four, and Cletus is almost three."

After I asked Mrs. Crummett when her children had first gotten sick, she gazed at me in bewilderment, like I had asked her to recite the Gettysburg Address. "I don't really know. Sometime last week, I guess."

"Have they been to see a doctor about this problem?"

Mrs. Crummett told me that several weeks earlier, a Health Department doctor had prescribed a pink liquid medicine for the twins. At the time, they had seemed to improve, but for the last two nights, they hadn't slept well. She then added uneasily that the Health Department doctor was off on Thursdays.

"You probably haven't slept much either," I said.

Mrs. Crummett nodded. Since her construction worker husband stayed in North Carolina for five days each week, she was caring for the children single-handedly.

Simple Gifts

Thinking about my own four children, I wondered how long I would survive as a single parent. Not very long, I decided.

"It will just take a few minutes to check your twins," I said, fastening a disposable plastic speculum to my otoscope. "Maybe you can take off their jackets so I can listen to their lungs."

"Oh, I'll do that!" declared Dixie. Her dirty fingers hurried to unbutton two very soiled coats that were several sizes too big.

Probably picks up their clothes in a thrift shop, I mused as I looked at the angry red bulges that had replaced glistening gray eardrums.

"Both Iris and Loretta have ear infections," I announced, adding that I would prescribe a Medicaid-approved antibiotic for each of them.

Mrs. Crummett promised to start the medicine that afternoon. Then shifting her gaze away from me, she looked at Dixie and Cletus. "Doctor, can you check the other two while we're here today? I think they're starting to get it too."

Anger erupted in my chest. Would I never get out of this stifling room? Then I looked again at the olive green discharge that was dripping onto Cletus's gray sweatshirt. "Okay, we'll work them in."

When I told Ellen that I needed two more new office charts, her hazel eyes blazed. After dictating short notes on Iris and Loretta, I spent several minutes at the lab faucet, scrubbing my hands with hot water and antiseptic soap.

Reentering the exam room, I braked so abruptly that my shoes squeaked on the tiles. Iris and Loretta were using several dozen wooden tongue blades to construct a plank road that led from the exam table to the corner sink. Dixie had inflated four plastic gloves to create balloons for Cletus, who was bouncing his new toys off the ceiling. As passive as a marble statue, Mrs. Crummett gazed out the window.

"Well, I see you kids have been busy," I managed. Stepping over the roadbuilding project, I advanced toward my next two patients. "Let's check you out so that you can go home and play."

Go home, I thought hopefully as I listened to their chests, *home where you can play outside in the fresh air.*

"Dixie and Cletus have bronchitis," I said to Mrs. Crummett. Writing two more prescriptions, I noted that the twins needed to be rechecked in two weeks.

"You can all get dressed now," I said to the children. "Ellen probably has some suckers for you."

With a whoop, Dixie leaped off the exam table. "Suckers!" she exclaimed to her siblings. "We're going to get suckers!"

As our dingy procession moved down the hall, Ellen met us with the lollipops and a roll of adhesive cartoon stickers. Lathering up with more antiseptic soap, I heard a chorus of excited voices. "I want Mickey Mouse! No, Donald Duck for me!"

"Well, at least they left happy," Ellen remarked.

"And courtesy of those happy children, you're facing quite a clean-up job."

Picking up an aerosol can of industrial strength Lysol, Ellen headed down the hall. In a moment, she was back, her face flaming. "You didn't tell me that I'd have to restock everything too. What were you all doing in there, playing hospital?"

Buried in another chart, I mumbled something about being thankful that the Crummetts wouldn't be back for two more weeks and that surely by that time, they would have had their monthly baths.

In both of my assumptions, I was completely wrong. In only four days, the Crummetts reappeared, en famille and more aromatic than ever.

"How could they do this on a Monday afternoon?" Ellen raged.

"How could they do it on any day?" I retorted as I headed down the hall.

"And how is everyone this afternoon?" I asked as I breached the outer defenses of cotton balls and Q-tips. "I thought you were coming back next week."

Mrs. Crummett looked dazed. "I think maybe they're getting better, but I wanted you to recheck them."

After my examination, I shared Mrs. Crummett's assessment and asked her to continue all present treatment. She nodded. "And I need a new diaper for Cletus. That antibiotic has given him some bad diarrhea."

On Cletus's jumpsuit, mustard yellow stains caught my eye. So that was the exotic new ingredient in today's fragrance. "No problem, Mrs. Crummett. The nurse will bring you a clean diaper."

"And then we'll get our suckers and stickers!" rejoiced Dixie.

In spite of everything, I smiled.

That evening, Ellen presented her solution. "So the Crummetts are coming back again next week?"

I nodded.

"You do know they're from Greene County, don't you? I don't see why the Greene County doctors can't care for their own welfare patients!"

By Ellen's lights, it was possible that something good might come out of Nazareth but never out of Greene County.

"Well, there's no law that tells Medicaid patients where to go for medical care," I countered. "Where do you think the Crummetts should go?"

"To the University Pediatric Clinic. That's what the state has its clinics for—to take care of people like the Crummetts." Looking directly at me, she delivered her knockout. "And do you know, Dr. J., that Medicaid only pays us $7.00 for each office visit?"

I winced. In 1986, $7.00 was less than half of our regular office fee. Because of meager reimbursement, most area doctors did not see Medicaid patients. Like so many other government health programs, the Medicaid system penalized both the patients and the physicians.

Ellen pushed on. "I think that each Crummett probably costs us $7.00 just in clean-up bills. After all, Dr. J., supplies aren't free—tongue blades, cotton balls, Lysol, diapers . . ."

I gulped.

"Exam gloves, stickers, suckers," she continued, her eyes drilling into mine.

"Well, I don't know," I vacillated, envisioning a single mother driving to Charlottesville every time her children got sick.

In the tone that she saved for my most pigheaded moments, Ellen asked me to just think about it.

The next ten January days—crammed with pneumonia, influenza, and strep throat—raced by like a movie film on fast forward. When Ellen once more handed me the four Crummett charts, I stared at her in disbelief.

"Did they walk in again?" I asked. My fuse was smoking.

"Oh, no! They're blue ink patients today. This is the ear recheck for the twins." Then polishing her one-of-a-kind engagement ring, Ellen added that Mrs. Crummett also wanted me to check Dixie and Cletus.

Looking at the two extra charts, I snarled. "And how is everyone today?"

"Oh, much better! Their temperatures are all normal, and nobody's coughing, at least, not very much." Ellen tapped the charts on my desktop. "And I talked to Mrs. Crummett about keeping the kids out of the supply drawers. This time when they got here, I gave them a big box of crayons and some paper."

I grunted.

"And there's one more thing that you'll notice right away. They've finally had their monthly baths!"

"Really!" I looked up from my desk. This news brief had snagged my attention. "Why do you suppose that happened?"

Ellen ventured that it was probably because Mr. Crummett was back home again. Fortunately, his job in North Carolina had gone well, and he had been reassigned to a new project within easy commuting distance.

Even with Ellen's reassurance, I sniffed before filling my lungs with normal exam room air.

"And how are the Crummetts this afternoon?" I asked as I surveyed a quartet of industrious artists.

"I think they're all better," said Mrs. Crummett. Today she looked completely different. What a smile and some lipstick can do for a certain type of woman is nothing short of miraculous.

"The twins' ears are fine," I reported as I finished my examination. "Of course, at their age, they're really prone to ear infections. If they do start running a fever again, you should bring them back to the office right away."

Appalled by my slipup, I made a midcourse correction. "What I meant to say is that you should call and make an appointment. We'll be glad to see you the same day."

With a shy smile, Mrs. Crummett said that she understood.

After checking Cletus's lungs, which were as clear as a summer day, I knelt beside the little girl who was polishing the fine points of her artwork. Dixie's lungs were normal too. "Can I see your drawing?" I asked.

The artist added two more green lines before laying down her crayon. "Oh, I drew my picture for you!" she said with a grin.

I leaned over to admire her gift.

"Do you know who that is?" my little patient asked, giggling.

"I think so," I said. The crayon drawing was graced with the charm of a child's work. In the center, a tall angular man wore a long white coat, complete with a malformed stethoscope. His smile—a scarlet half-moon—neatly bisected his face while uniting the blue circles of his ears. His jade green eyes were dysconjugate but happy. From his coat pockets peeped a collection of lollipops—red, purple, green, and gold.

On the left side of the drawing, an equally long-limbed nurse boasted an orange smile that was just as wide as the doctor's. Black corkscrews of hair hung to her waist, and multicolored circles decorated her uniform.

"That's a picture of my nurse and me, isn't it?" I asked softly. "Dixie, you're a real artist!"

My patient's smile was almost as broad as those of her creations.

"Keeping suckers in my pocket is a really good idea," I continued. "Now I can have a snack whenever I want one."

Dixie giggled.

"But just one thing," I said, pointing to the colorful spots on Ellen's lab suit. "What are all these things that look like Christmas balls?"

Dixie doubled over with laughter. "They're not Christmas balls. Those are stickers! Can't you tell?"

I agreed that, without a doubt, that's exactly what they were and walked with the Crummetts out of the exam room. When we reached my cubicle, I tore off three strips of surgical tape, and Dixie, standing on tiptoe, taped her masterpiece to my door.

"And now it's time for suckers and stickers!" the little girl said as she smiled at Iris, Loretta, and Cletus. "I can hardly wait!"

As I was dictating their charts, Ellen appeared in the doorway. I switched off my recorder.

"The Crummetts are checking out now," she said, "and I need to know if I should refer them to the Pediatric Clinic."

"No, you won't need to do that."

"Are you sure you feel that way? They do have Medicaid, you know."

I shook my head. "Ellen, from the economic angle, you're certainly right, but I'm actually looking forward to taking care of them."

Suppressing her common sense, my nurse turned away. Leaning over, I touched her elbow.

"Just one more thing," I said, pointing to the crayon picture that was brightening my door.

Ellen's eyes softened.

"That's a picture of you and me," I said. "Dixie gave that to me just now, and I've always been partial to beginning artists."

CHAPTER TWELVE

HEALTH-CARE DELIVERY BY BULLDOZER

> Stories are medicine. I have been taken with stories since I heard my first. They have such power; they do not require that we do, be, act anything—we need only listen.
> —Clarissa Estes, *Women Who Run With the Wolves*

"Eight inches of snow, and it's still coming down!"

Doreen was excited as she pulled off her boots and parka. After flying down the back hill with our four children on the toboggan, we had all come inside for hot chocolate.

"The weatherman says we'll get a foot," I commented, adding my icy gloves to the collection of winter clothes that was drying near our woodstove. "And this time I think he's right on target."

On this gray Saturday morning, the first flakes had drifted down during office hours, and by the time our last patient had left at noon, two inches of soft new snow blanketed the landscape. Driving homeward on Route 29—Madison's solitary four-lane highway—I saw only a few tractor-trailers. Apparently, most people had believed the weatherman and were staying home.

By the time I reached County Road 631, the snow was falling with renewed determination. Several savvy neighbors had parked their four-wheel drive pickups near the junction of Route 29 and our winding county road. Recognizing precaution that was born of experience, I angled my truck beside theirs, pulled on my hiking boots, and started the two-mile jaunt to our house.

When County Road 631 was laid out during Virginia's colonial era, the original construction crew apparently cared little for the notion that the shortest distance between two points is a straight line. Our road wanders over hills and crisscrosses meadows as if to flaunt its own inefficiency. Flowing lazily beside the road is an equally impractical stream—aptly named Crooked Run. Today its shallow pools were iced over and covered with snow.

As I puffed up the last hill, our four children spotted me and screamed with delight. Soon we had all piled onto the toboggan and were racing down the back hill into the orchard. And now with a steaming cup of hot chocolate, it felt good to relax by a crackling fire and to listen to a contented tea kettle.

"I think I'll fix vegetable soup for dinner," Doreen said. She was enjoying our family afternoon at home. "And how about some cornbread to go along with it?"

"Sounds wonderful." Leaning back into the recliner, I put my feet up and reached down to stroke our yellow cat, Oliver. Inside our house, it was so cozy, and outside around the white pine trees, the snow swirled down in such soothing rhythms.

When the phone jangled, I jumped.

"Hello," I said, shaking off the remnants of my afternoon nap.

"Doc, this is Rob Thorson," a familiar voice said. "Sorry to bother you at home, but I wondered if you could help me out with a squad call?"

I asked what was happening. Only rarely did the local volunteer rescue squad contact me after office hours. Usually, they transported their patients directly to the University Hospital.

"It's Myra Collins," Rob began. "She's having another asthma attack, and I'm concerned that we may not be able to get her to Charlottesville in this storm. I can pick you up at your house in my ATV."

"I'll be ready when you get here," I said.

As I climbed back into my snowsuit and ski cap, I tried to remember the details of Myra Collins's single office visit. I recalled an elderly woman—underweight, brown hair streaked with gray, a hesitant gait, anxious eyes. Usually, she saw a pulmonary physician at the University.

When Rob pulled into our driveway, snow was falling steadily in the beams of the headlights. "I'll be home for dinner," I promised as I kissed Doreen good-bye.

"No rush," said my amiable spouse "The refrigerator isn't working exactly right, so I'm going to replace the motor." Anticipation glowed in the eyes of our resident mechanic.

I wished her well. The soup smelled wonderful as I stepped out into a frozen world.

Rob was an expert driver, but his ATV slipped a few times on the twists and turns of County Road 631. Finally, we were southbound on Route 29. In the early twilight, highway crews were fighting to keep a single lane of the main highway open. Even the tractor-trailers had disappeared.

"Doc, Myra Collins rings us up almost every time it snows." Rob sprayed the grimy windshield with deicer fluid. "She lives by herself, and I think she gets nervous in bad weather."

I commented that her calls must make the paramedic's snow days just that much more hectic. Rob nodded. Even if Mrs. Collins needed to go to the hospital this time, he wasn't sure he could get her there in this winter storm.

"Well, let's hope she doesn't need to go," I said.

Replying that we would know in a few minutes, Rob turned off the highway and into the snow-filled lane of a country house. Spinning on the unplowed driveway, we finally reached the white frame residence. Tall magnolia trees, their dark leaves heavy with snow, bordered the long wraparound porch. Together, Rob and I stomped up to the front door.

I recognized Myra Collins at once. Although she was dressed in a quilted plaid housecoat, she was still the same small-featured elderly lady that I had seen in our office. Without any cosmetics, her face was pale. Her thin nose held up a green oxygen cannula.

Mrs. Collins told me that she had gotten worse just this morning and that she had completed three nebulizer treatments. As I checked her lungs, I heard only scattered wheezes. There were no sounds to suggest pneumonia, and her heart was strong and regular.

"I'd like to see the medicines that you've been taking," I said.

From the marble-top bedside table, Mrs. Collins lifted a carved wooden sewing box. As I raised the lid, Rob's pager went off.

Consternation spread across the paramedic's bearded face. "There's been a truck accident, Doc, and I need to leave right away. Can you stay here with Mrs. Collins? I'll come back as soon as I can."

I looked at Mrs. Collins wary eyes. "Of course," I agreed. "We'll be okay until you get back."

Rob's running footsteps receded down the hall, and the front door slammed. Glancing at Myra Collins, I tilted her sewing box and filled a corner of the bedspread with medication bottles.

"Well, let's go through these first," I proposed. Here, for a start, was a project that should keep us occupied for quite a while.

To begin with, there were three aerosol inhalers, two bottles of cough syrup, and a container of nasal spray. Many of the pill bottles were empty, and I separated them from the full ones. This winnowing process still left eighteen bottles—medications for asthma, arthritis, pain, indigestion, dizziness, anxiety, and insomnia. Opening her bedside table drawer, Mrs. Collins added two bottles of antibiotic capsules to our home pharmacy.

"Mrs. Collins, you use several medications." I have always enjoyed an understatement. "How do you keep them all straight?"

Mrs. Collins explained that she didn't use everything every day. Her pulmonary physician encouraged her to keep extra supplies of her medicines on hand so that she could modify her treatment regimen whenever her symptoms flared.

"What seems to trigger your asthma attacks?"

Mrs. Collins told me that a variety of factors aggravated her condition. Upper respiratory infections always caused her to wheeze, and twice in the past year, she had been hospitalized for pneumonia. She was also allergic to dust, molds, maple pollen, ragweed, and summer grasses.

"And last year, I had to give away my two Persian cats," she continued. Her eyes were sad. "I'd had them for years, but my asthma doctor insists that I can't keep any pets. I still miss my cats. They were such a lot of company."

I thought about our yellow Oliver, sleeping by the stove at home. "Pets are good friends."

"I don't have any close neighbors, Doctor. In fact, I don't get many visitors anymore. Of course, Lydia comes in on weekdays. She's the housekeeper and does all the cleaning and cooking. But usually on weekends, I'm here by myself."

When I asked about her family, Mrs. Collins shook her head. Two elderly cousins lived in the next county, but neither of them drove anymore. My patient rarely took her own car out. She was afraid of the speeding tractor-trailers on Route 29.

"And Celia, my daughter, lives in Texas," Mrs. Collins continued. Celia was the headmistress of a girls' school, and her husband was an attorney. Celia's work schedule was so demanding that she hadn't been back to Virginia for several years. She had never had any children.

"We don't get together for Christmas anymore," Mrs. Collins informed me. "It's just too complicated. I used to fly to Texas every December, but since my health's been failing, it's just easier to stay home."

I thought about this elderly lady all alone in a large country house at Christmas. "Have you lived here a long time, Mrs. Collins?"

"Practically all my life, Doctor." In fact, she had been born in an upstairs bedroom and had spent her childhood here. After high school, she had completed two years of teacher's training but had never actually worked as a schoolteacher. Just before World War II broke out, she had married an army intelligence officer. A year later, he had been killed in the blitz bombing of London, and two months after that, Celia had been born.

When Mrs. Collins paused, her eyes were far away from Madison.

After her husband's death, she had moved back to her childhood home, and she had been here ever since. Both of her parents had died in this house—her father quite suddenly from a heart attack and her mother ten years later after a protracted struggle with bone cancer. By that time, Celia was married and gone, and Mrs. Collins had lived here alone.

"This house has been in our family for five generations," she said, reflecting. "But of course, all that will end when I'm gone. Celia won't ever come back to Madison to live. She loves Texas and plans to stay there when she retires."

Behind me, the mantel clock chimed the hour—6:00. I rechecked my patient's lungs. They sounded almost normal.

"Let's see how you feel off the oxygen," I suggested. Mrs. Collins nodded, and I slipped off her cannula and closed the valve on the oxygen tank.

"Your home must have a lot of memories for you," I said.

Mrs. Collins's face softened. "Seventy-four years of memories." Her hands toyed with the border of her afghan as she talked about old times.

There was the Christmas when her father had built a dollhouse for her out in the toolshed and had brought it into the parlor on a festive December morning. There had been her mother's flower garden with its perennial border of hollyhocks, foxglove, and larkspur. And there had been her family's first car. She laughed a little as she recalled the black Model A Ford that had broken down on its maiden voyage. Her father was bringing it home from town, and he had to finish his trip on a horse. And of course, there had been her little brother, laughing as he slid down the staircase banister into the waiting arms of his big sister.

"I didn't realize that you had a brother."

Mrs. Collins looked at the snow-covered windowpanes. "Billy died when he was only five years old. He caught the measles and died a week later, right here in this very room." She pointed to the oval frame of an old-fashioned photograph hanging on the wall. The faded black-and-white print and the lace collar were grossly mismatched with the freckles and mischievous eyes of a young boy.

"You know," Mrs. Collins observed, "I think that ever since Billy died, this house has always felt a little lonesome."

I nodded. When I was seven, my baby sister had died, and after that, our house had never been the same. Withdrawing into his own darkness, my father had really never come out again.

"Billy died just two days before Christmas. It was a blizzard that year, and we couldn't get him to the cemetery for over a week. We kept the coffin here in the parlor for all that time." Mrs. Collins's eyes were haunted. "And after all these years, it's still a lot harder whenever it snows."

In silence, we sat together, remembering the loss of our childhood innocence—sudden, devastating, and irrevocable.

Mrs. Collins was the first to speak. "Well, I'm definitely breathing better, and if I'm not mistaken, I hear the Rescue Squad trying to get back up my lane."

Above the ticking of the clock, I heard it too—the sounds of a truck spinning, backing up, spinning again, and finally stopping right outside the front porch.

"I think you're going to be okay," I said. "Certainly, you'll want to keep up your nebulizer treatments, but you don't need to go to the hospital."

In the doorway, Rob's face brightened. "That's great news, Doc! The snow has slowed down, but it's a real mess out there. Only twenty degrees and the wind's getting up. We need to get you home before the drifts get too high."

I said good-bye to Mrs. Collins, who agreed to call me if she had any more problems with her asthma.

As Rob and I slid down her driveway, Route 29 was much worse than when we had arrived two hours before. Only a few snowflakes were still falling, but an Arctic wind was piling up drifts with amazing efficiency.

Just ahead of us on the highway, the flashing yellow lights of a Virginia Transportation Department bulldozer hurled circles of light out into the darkness.

"There's your ride home, Doc!" Rob announced cheerfully. "With a storm like this, there's no way that I can get my ATV anywhere on County Road 631, but that's my cousin on the dozer, and he says he'll be sure to get you home."

Grabbing my medical bag, I hoisted myself up into the tractor cab behind the burly driver. As I held onto the metal frame, the dozer started off with a jerk. Around the curves and through the snowdrifts of our county road, I was going home on a bulldozer.

Above the roar of the diesel engine and the clack of the metal tracks, I enjoyed the shouted comment of my chauffeur. "Doc, if you keep riding around like this, you're going to be another Dr. Rucker! Nothing ever stopped her either!"

Holding onto the swaying cab, I felt a rush of elation like a glass of red wine on an empty stomach. Here I was, a hometown doctor, making house calls by bulldozer and reminding someone of my legendary predecessor. Above the blizzard, the gods were smiling.

Cupping my gloved hands together, I welcomed the compliment. "Glad to hear you say so, sir. That next driveway on the right will be our house. And many thanks. This is a great way to travel!"

CHAPTER THIRTEEN

HEARTBREAK ON WALKER'S BOTTOM ROAD

> **All flesh is as grass, and all the glory of man as the flower of grass. The grass withereth, and the flower thereof falleth away.**
> —1 Peter 1:24

❧

"Doc, are you the coroner this evening?" Paramedic Rob Thorson's deep voice was urgent. After office hours, he had tracked me down at one of my never-ending side jobs—my war of attrition with medical paperwork.

"You've got your man, Rob." Several evenings each month, I was the backup medical examiner for Madison County, while Dr. Samuels and his wife went bowling. "What's going on?"

"It's a bad accident, Doc. A sports car hit a tree on Walker's Bottom Road. Only one kid in the car, but he's dead as a doornail. Just need you to make it official."

"I'll be right there, Rob. Are the police on the scene?"

"No, but they're on their way, should get here about the same time you do. We're on Walker's Bottom Road, about half a mile east of Walker's Church." Rob's tone changed. "Now don't you drive too fast, Doc. The roads are really icy out here tonight."

Grabbing my medical examiner's bag, I walked out into a frigid February night. Covering the parking lot was a thick layer of ice that softened in the daytime only to become rock-hard again after sundown.

Driving slowly along the winding county roads, I was surrounded by a Currier and Ives landscape. Over the eastern horizon hovered a full orange moon that outlined the homes, barns, and fencerows of sleeping dairy farms. Near the roadside, a flock of black and white Canadian geese roosted by a frozen pond.

Just past Walker's Church, the pastoral peace ended. A constellation of flashing lights—red, yellow, and blue—lit up the adjacent pasture fields. Adding my truck to the line of emergency service vehicles by the highway, I spotted Rob Thorson's giant frame. In his snowsuit, he was more massive than ever.

"Glad you got here okay, Doc," Rob said, greeting me. The accident had happened forty minutes ago, but the paramedic had spent a frustrating half-hour trying to track down Dr. Samuels. Together, we walked toward the red flares and a somber state policeman.

"This poor kid hit the tree head-on," Rob explained, pointing toward a gigantic maple tree. At the base of its triple trunk was a crumpled silver sports car. "Probably was going way too fast and tried to brake on the ice."

I nodded. In the hills of Madison County, Walker's Bottom Road's singularly straight stretch of highway offered tempting opportunities for local daredevils. On any clear day, the skid marks testified to the road's reputation, but tonight, its surface was a sheen of ice.

Stepping carefully over a drainage ditch, I saw the classic lines of a new Jaguar—an engineering marvel with chrome and horsepower to spare. The front end looked like a giant hammer had smashed it.

Avoiding shards of broken glass, I peered through the shattered windshield. Slumped over the steering wheel was a youthful body, still tethered by its waist and shoulder restraints. Like a rag doll tossed carelessly aside, the pale motionless face lay at a crazy angle. This driver had died instantly when his cervical spine had snapped, crushing his upper spinal cord.

After I authorized the extrication of the body, an EMT crew pried open the car door. Working as gently as parents moving a sleeping child, they eased the body onto the stretcher. Under the glare of the spotlights, the beardless face looked impossibly young. The boy probably weighed less than 120 pounds.

The policeman shuffled through the contents of a brown wallet. "It looks like this young man is, or should I say was, Chris Wyse. He's sixteen years old. Got his driver's license on his last birthday, November 20."

Listening to a spate of identifying information, I jotted a few notes on the margin of the medical examiner's form. Until tonight, this boy and I had been strangers, but now we were suddenly intimates. I was his final physician—the doctor designated by the state to investigate and certify the circumstances of a violent death.

Carefully palpating the torso and limbs of a still-pliable body, I found no injuries except the cervical spine fracture-dislocation. No ribs were broken; his abdomen—still warm—was flat; and his skull was intact. Opening a padded manila envelope, I extracted a large vacutainer syringe with a fourteen-gauge needle.

"Let's get the toxicology samples, Rob," I said.

Kneeling on the frozen sod, the paramedic watched as I used Betadine to prep the skin over the victim's left jugular vein. When Rob positioned the boy's head, both of us heard and felt the crunch of fractured vertebrae. The paramedic looked at me and shook his bearded head.

As I punctured the vein, dark red blood spurted into the vacuum tubes. Although a huge majority of fatal teenage accidents are triggered by alcohol and drug abuse, I somehow felt that Chris Wyse would be the exception. Inside his car, there had been no beer cans, and I couldn't smell any alcohol on the body. Carefully labeling the state's evidence, I placed it in the designated Styrofoam container and slipped it into my coat pocket.

"The next of kin has a local address," the policeman remarked. "Maureen Wyse resides here in Madison, Virginia." A frown settled over his lined forehead. "In all this rotten business, here's the part that I hate the most—having to go tell the mother."

Inside the warm woolen lining of my parka, I shivered. As the father of two teenage sons, I didn't want to think about opening my front door to confront a stone-faced police officer.

"I know where Mrs. Wyse lives," Rob Thorson said to the policeman. "Doc and I had better go with you this time."

The paramedic then explained that Mrs. Wyse was a widow and that Chris was an only child. Several years ago, her husband, an Air Force colonel, had been critically injured in a plane crash. About a year later, he had died at home. Mrs. Wyse now divided her time between her Madison County estate and her vacation home at St. Simon's Island.

After the body was loaded into the ambulance for its long ride to the state morgue in Richmond, and after the tow truck arrived, the policeman said that we were ready to leave the scene. Our convoy of three vehicles—the cruiser, Rob's ATV, and my pickup—wound slowly up Walker's Bottom Road, made a number of turns, and finally climbed a long private driveway to reach the Wyse residence. A stately antebellum home, it crowned a wooded knoll that overlooked the Robinson River.

A servant, a middle-aged woman, opened the front door. Her terrified eyes told me immediately that she had guessed everything. Within seconds, we three visitors were seated in a spacious reception room, awaiting the arrival of Mrs. Wyse. Across from me, hanging above a carved mantel, was an oil painting of a handsome young Air Force officer. Its gold leaf frame matched the pattern of the room's crown molding.

Thirty minutes later, when I was climbing back into my truck, the preceding scene still dominated me completely. The horror on Maureen Wyse's face, the solitary scream that escaped her contoured lips, and the sobs that racked her slim body would be part of me for the rest of my life. She had accepted my offer of a prescription for sleeping pills, but we both recognized this for what it was—a polite but futile gesture.

By the next morning, our entire community shared my shock. In fact, no one talked of anything else. Chris Wyse had been the president of his high school junior class, and the tragic death of this gifted student and star basketball player tapped into the deepest emotions of everyone who knew him. The funeral, scheduled for Saturday, would be at the Madison Methodist Church, where Mrs. Wyse was an inactive member.

My oldest son, one of Chris's classmates, kept his eyes on the floor as he informed me about the cancellation of Friday's basketball game.

Every church organist owns the best seat in the house. Arriving early on Saturday with a sheaf of funeral music, I watched a multitude of solemn Madisonians find their seats on the crowded pews. Soon, the overflow had filled the foyer and was spilling out into the churchyard.

Just before noon, I caught the funeral director's signal and lifted my fingers from the keyboard. Changing the setting of the stops, I began the soft melancholy chords of Verdi's *Requiem*. "Grant them rest, grant them rest, grant them Thy eternal reset."

Back in the foyer, there was a stir, and the congregation—united in an expression of respect—stood. Escorted by the funeral director, Maureen Wyse walked to the front of the church, kissed the coffin covered with white roses, and sat. A handful of relatives, all in mourning dress, soon joined her.

Simple Gifts

Under my fingers, Verdi's venerable notes came to life. "For Thou art good, Thou art good. Grant them rest, grant them rest. Gentle Jesus, gentle Jesus, grant them thy eternal rest."

Finally, the requiem ended, the congregation sat, and the short pallid Methodist minister walked hesitantly to his pulpit. In all of his ecclesiastical appearances, the Reverend Wes Weebley was unsure of himself, but today he was more awkward than ever. With thick glasses riveted to his Book of Common Prayer, he monotoned the standard Protestant funeral service: the Lord is gracious and full of compassion; the Lord will satisfy his children with abundant mercy; the one true God—almighty and everlasting—has been pleased to take unto himself the soul of our departed brother.

After a recitation of God's inscrutable attributes, Reverend Weebley closed his book and offered a nondescript prayer. As he sat down, he looked more than usually out of place. Perhaps there are no politically correct things to say at the funeral of a teenager.

Following a recessional and a slow drive across town to the cemetery, we were all together once more, huddled against the keen winter wind that ripped at the green awnings of the funeral tent. After the Wyse family was escorted to the folding chairs beside the open grave, Reverend Weebley recited some more inaudible rubric and then looked at the funeral director.

The funeral director nodded and raised his hand. From the hillside to our left came the discordance of brass instruments tuning up. Standing on tiptoe, I saw the high school band in parade formation.

The conductor raised her baton, and all around us flowed the simple melody and harmony of "Amazing Grace." Through the cypress and holly trees, the plaintive notes rose, lingered, fell, and then died away.

With a growing lump in my throat, I stared down at the dead turf. Somehow I really didn't want to look up to see the pathetic figure of Reverend Weebley attempting a benediction.

Suddenly, a baritone voice rang through the cemetery. "Friends, it's time for all of us to pray together."

In surprise, I looked up to see Mark Detamore, the pastor of the Deep Run Baptist Church, standing by the funeral director. As Mark raised his muscular arms, his Southern drawl echoed through the crowd.

"Our heavenly Father, we come to you today in grief of soul. From beyond the reach of our loving arms has gone our friend, yes, and more than our friend, our son, Chris Wyse."

As Mark paused, I heard the soft weeping of first one person, and then another, and then many more. Except for the restless wind, our sobs were the only sounds in the cemetery.

I was deaf to the rest of my Baptist friend's words. Just now, I only had room for my own feelings—my grief for Chris Wyse, for his mother, and for the frail mortality shared by us all. But in the Baptist minister's prayer was a power and a pathos that were strangely comforting. His firm "Amen!" felt like an honest benediction.

I wiped my eyes in time to see Maureen Wyse make the first move. Rising from her folding chair, she walked over to Mark Detamore, started to say something, and then collapsed into his arms. I got misty again as I saw Mark hold Mrs. Wyse tightly to his chest and then walk with her back to the waiting funeral home Cadillac.

The post-funeral reception took place in the high school cafeteria. Our church social hall was hopelessly inadequate for the task at hand. As I mingled with the crowd, I spotted my mother talking with Aunt Lillian.

"Harold, I certainly enjoyed your organ music," Aunt Lillian said as she handed me a paper plate. "You'd better get yourself a slice of my lemon pound cake before it's all gone."

"Yes, you'd better," agreed my mother. "I haven't seen such a crowd at a funeral in many a long year."

"I was glad that the Baptist minister prayed in the cemetery," Aunt Lillian continued. "I'm sure we Methodists are fortunate to have Reverend Weebley, but he's not real good in an emergency, is he?" She bit into her ham biscuit. "Why, he's already gone back to the parsonage. Mrs. Weebley said that his sinuses always bother him after he is outside in the wind."

My mother showed little sympathy for her stricken minister. "I wouldn't ever want to be a Baptist myself, of course, but they all certainly are pleased with their new preacher, and after today I can see why."

Looking across the cafeteria, I saw Mark Detamore sitting beside Maureen Wyse. He was holding her hand.

"Yes, Mom," I said, nodding to one of the lasting authority figures in my life. "After today I can see why they are too."

CHAPTER FOURTEEN

OLD KNEES AND OLDER ANIMOSITIES

> **Doctors are just the same as lawyers; the only difference is that lawyers merely rob you, whereas doctors rob you and kill you, too.**
>
> —Anton Chekhov

"Doctor, it's so good to see you again!" The elderly African American woman's greeting brightened the functional space of the exam room. On this cloudy February day, her broad smile and sparkling black eyes were as warm as a Virginia summer.

"It's good to see you too, Mrs. Beasley," I said. "It's been a long time, hasn't it?"

Mrs. Beasley responded by stepping toward me and wrapping me in her big arms. I savored the bear hug.

"Well!" said Mrs. Beasley, stepping back to a more detached perspective. "I've never hugged a doctor before! And aren't you looking good, Harold! I'm glad to see that you've put on a few pounds since you were in school."

I laughed out loud. Only Mrs. Beasley could comment on my midwinter weight gain with such honest pleasure. Through my seven years of elementary education, I had been so underweight that my ribs stuck out like bumps under my T-shirts. As the school cook, Mrs. Beasley had viewed my scrawniness as a professional challenge.

While we students had chattered in the cafeteria line, the savory fragrance of beef stew or spaghetti or barbecue filled the air. And in front of us was Mrs. Beasley—splendid in a starched white uniform and a white hairnet—presiding over the steam table.

"Now, Harold, you eat all of that," she would command as she loaded my plate with hot food. "It's good for you!" Then her hearty laugh allowed a glimpse of the gold tooth—an appendage that always fascinated me.

I smiled at the memories. In the twenty-four years since I had been a Madison elementary student, Mrs. Beasley had both changed and remained the same. Her thick black hair was now heavily streaked with gray, but she still wore it in a big bun on the back of her neck. The horn-rimmed glasses and gold chain were new additions.

"Are you enjoying your retirement, Mrs. Beasley?"

"I certainly am. It's been really nice this winter to look out at all that ice and not go traipsing off to work. Now I just sit down and have another cup of coffee."

I told my patient that, given her inexhaustible energy level, she probably didn't linger too long over breakfast.

Mrs. Beasley ruefully patted her knees. "That's why I've come to see you, Harold. There are so many things that these old joints won't let me do." For at least ten years, she had experienced stiffness in her knees, especially in the mornings. At first, aspirin had been a big help, but now she felt some discomfort whenever she walked and especially when she descended a flight of stairs.

Over the years, Dr. Rucker had prescribed an array of anti-inflammatory medicines, but none had worked particularly well. "Doctor, I've probably just worn my legs out on that cement cafeteria floor. After all, I worked there for forty-six years, you know."

Looking at my patient, I thought about her odyssey—the thousands of miles that she had logged at the elementary school. "You may have a point there. Let's take a look at your knees."

When Mrs. Beasley stood, I spotted the carved wooden cane that was hooked over the back of her chair. My patient walked cautiously, and as she stepped up onto the footrest, she reached for my arm. Around her sizable legs, thick cables of varicose veins climbed like grapevines on an arbor. As I touched feet that were longer and broader than mine, I was relieved to feel the regular rhythm of normal arterial pulses.

When I palpated her knees, I understood why Mrs. Beasley used a cane. Her arthritic spurs were sharp and prominent, and when either joint moved, the associated grinding was audible.

"Your knees are talking to us today," I observed.

"And some days, I talk back to them, but usually, they have the last word." Mrs. Beasley laughed as she agreed to my suggestion of X-rays.

The message of her films was unmistakable. The wear and tear of time had essentially destroyed her knees. Dagger-sharp spurs surrounded her joint margins. After years of weight bearing, her cartilage had completely vanished, leaving bone to scrape against bone. Not even Mrs. Beasley's iron willpower would always be able to override the pathology that had taken up residence in her knees.

As I gave my patient a guided tour of her X-rays, she studied the films with interest. "So, Doctor, what do I need to do about all of this?"

Given the severity of her joint destruction, I doubted that any medicine would help for long. "You probably need knee replacement surgery."

"I was afraid that you would say that. So far, I've never had any operations, thank the good Lord, but if that's what I need, I'll get through it somehow." Mrs. Beasley looked at her films and hesitated. "But I do want to talk to my daughter first. Joyce is coming down from Washington this weekend."

I said that there was no need to hurry.

"Joyce always thinks of so many things that never occur to me." Mrs. Beasley's face glowed with maternal pride. "She's done so well for herself. She's got a good job in a great big law firm. I still wish that she had gotten married, but she says that this job is her life."

I told Mrs. Beasley that I would be in the office all week and invited her to call anytime.

Halfway through our Saturday morning office hours, Ellen appeared at my cubicle door. Across her tanned face was a knowing smirk. "So where on the schedule do you want me to put the Beasleys?"

Ellen is fond of rhetorical questions.

"Oh, tell them to come in at twelve thirty. I'll talk to them after morning office hours."

Two hours later, Mrs. Beasley greeted me with her trademark gold-tooth smile. "Doctor! It's so nice of you to talk to us this afternoon. And I'm glad that you're getting to meet my daughter, Joyce."

For a moment, I had the disconcerting sense of seeing double. Standing close to me was the Mrs. Beasley of four days ago with her gray hair and carved wooden cane. But just beyond her was the Mrs. Beasley of my school days—tall, sturdy, dark-skinned, and confident. Of course, I had never known our cook to wear a navy blue suit and scalloped silver earrings, but the resemblance was striking.

Only when the younger woman extended her hand did I sense the difference. "How are you, Dr. Jenkins? I'm Joyce Beasley. Perhaps you'd like to have my card." From her leather date book, she extracted a textured business card, which identified her as a paralegal with a prominent Washington law firm.

"It's nice to meet you," I said, slipping the card into my lab coat pocket.

In her organization and her energy, Joyce was a younger edition of her mother—minus the amiability. As my paralegal visitor talked on, our exchange of information became an uneasy compromise between a conversation and a deposition. After twenty minutes of interrogation and discovery, we had rather exhausted the status of Mrs. Beasley's knees. When Joyce asked me to recommend a hospital for her mother, I suggested the University of Virginia.

Joyce frowned. "As I told Mother this morning, I prefer the Georgetown University Hospital. I'm working on my law degree there. Their department is especially strong in civil rights litigation."

Before I could agree that Georgetown would be just fine, my patient cut us off. "Now, Joyce, you know that I don't want to go anywhere in Washington. I never have liked all that rush and racket."

Joyce cleared her throat. "To be frank, Mother, I'm concerned that you may not receive the best possible medical care down here in Virginia." She gazed coolly at me. "Unfortunately for Mother, she's an elderly black woman on Medicare, and the American medical system is owned and operated by wealthy white men."

"Joyce!" There was steel in Mrs. Beasley's voice. "How can you say such a thing to Dr. Jenkins! Why, I've known him since he was in elementary school."

"I'm sure that you have, Mother. But that was an all-white school, wasn't it? When I came along, I couldn't go to that school, so I never really had the chance to meet Dr. Jenkins or any of your other white friends. And the only reason you know them, Mother, is because you've slaved for them every day of your life."

Simple Gifts

In the old cook's eyes, lightning flashed and thunder rolled. If ever an avenging Zeus had wanted to appear as a black female, he would have been well represented by Mrs. Beasley.

"Joyce," she said, gripping her cane, "that is more than enough! Why, I'm so embarrassed that I wish I had never come out here today. Doctor, you'll just have to excuse my daughter for the way she's acting."

As I remembered the era of racial segregation, with the shabby secondhand buses and dilapidated schools that were relegated for the black children, I looked down at the carpet. Joyce had many valid reasons for her anger.

"Why, there's nothing to excuse, Mrs. Beasley," I said. "Your daughter feels just like I did before my own mother had her knee replacement two years ago. Back then, I wanted to be sure that Mom got the very best available care." I smiled at my patient. "And I hope my kids will feel the same way when I get my knees replaced."

Mrs. Beasley propped her cane against the wall. "I hope it's a long time before either you or Joyce need this kind of surgery."

"Well," I said, "I've never been a school cook, but the way that I race around this office, I know I'll need new knees eventually." I gave my joints a proprietary pat. "It's just a matter of time!"

Mrs. Beasley laughed, and Joyce managed a smile. When she smiled, she looked so much better—so much more like her mother.

Since I had been pleased with my own mother's operation, I suggested that Mrs. Beasley see the same surgeon. Dr. Esther Wu, a friend of mine from medical school days, was now a top orthopedist at the University.

"I'm sure she'll be just fine," declared Mrs. Beasley. Joyce nodded. I agreed to arrange the appointment and to call my patient after I received Dr. Wu's consultation note.

"So it's all settled, thank the good Lord!" exclaimed Mrs. Beasley, picking up her cane. "Now if you two will excuse me, I just have to find the bathroom. This blood pressure pill keeps me going all the time."

As she disappeared around the corner, the paralegal and I walked out to the empty waiting room. "Joyce, I'm glad you could come in today," I said. "I've always enjoyed your mother."

"And I'm glad that you're her doctor. Of course, I wish that she wasn't living down here in the country all by herself, but I'll never convince her to move. She's absolutely bullheaded about doing everything her own way."

I looked at the paralegal's strong jaw.

"And I suspect that you and I are a lot like that, ourselves," I said. "If law school is anything like medical school, stubbornness is a person's most valuable asset."

Joyce grinned like I was a long-lost comrade. "Maybe we Madisonians are just naturally good at being obstinate."

Slowly, the bathroom door opened, and the three of us walked out to the parking lot. Joyce unlocked her blue BMW and helped Mrs. Beasley into the passenger seat.

"Mrs. Beasley, I'll contact Dr. Wu on Monday and then call you back when I get the consultation note."

Joyce added, "Mother can call me if she has any questions."

"Oh, I'll be calling you too," I said. "I think it would be helpful if the three of us stayed in contact."

"Now you don't have to do that, Doctor." The tone of Joyce's objection told me that she loved the idea.

Reaching into my lab coat, I fished out her business card. "No problem. I already have your telephone number."

Joyce's smile was collegial. "Okay! Talk to you soon!"

CHAPTER FIFTEEN

ELLA MAE BLOSSOM GOES TO STAUNTON

> **Human kind cannot bear very much reality.**
> —T. S. Eliot, *Murder in the Cathedral*

"Dr. J., I just had the most wonderful lunch!" In Ellen's voice was more than a hint of malice. Buried in paperwork and worried about my expanding waistline, I had passed up a trip to Umstadler's Restaurant and, sitting nobly at my desk, had eaten one small Granny Smith apple.

"The roast beef was perfect," she added as she hung up her coat. "And the lemon meringue pie wasn't bad either."

My stomach growled rebelliously.

"And I found you another patient at Umstadler's," Ellen continued. "Ella Mae Blossom is coming in."

"What's happening with Ella Mae?" Over the past few months, this middle-aged social worker had come into our office regularly to have her lithium levels checked. Sometimes I adjusted her dosage, but usually, I just forwarded a copy of my office note to the psychiatrist that managed her bipolar disorder.

"I think she's stopped taking her pills. You should have seen how she was carrying on at Umstadler's." Concern softened Ellen's voice. "I've known Ella Mae for a long time, and she's traveled some rough roads along the way. Why, she's been over at Staunton any number of times."

Simple Gifts

I nodded. Sixty-five miles from Madison, the small city of Staunton was home to our regional state psychiatric hospital. When a local citizen required inpatient psychiatric care, his family politely avoided any direct reference to the hospital and instead stated that their relative had "gone to Staunton." Every Madisonian sensed the world of meaning behind this coded statement.

"Well, we'll just have to see how things are when Ella Mae gets here," I said.

When she arrived, I knew immediately how things were. I was freezing some warts with liquid nitrogen when a door slammed with such force that both my patient and I jumped from our seats. Quickly finishing my assault on the papillomaviruses, I hurried off in the direction of boisterous laughter.

"I'd better go in now and help Ellen out," I decided.

My patient hailed me as her messiah. "Oh, Dr. Jenkins! I'm so glad to see you!" Ella Mae was sweating and panting like a distance runner. "Tell your nurse to stop hurting me!"

"I'm sorry you're not feeling well, Ella Mae."

My patient asserted that she had never felt better in her entire life.

"Well, let's check your blood pressure anyhow just to be sure." I looked at boldly frosted hair, bronze hoop earrings, and a dress that featured giant red and yellow tulips. On her previous visits, Ella Mae's face had been sedately middle-aged, but today, under layers of lipstick, rouge, and mascara, it seemed to be reaching desperately backward in time toward a youth that was forever gone.

Ellen peeled off the Velcro cuff. "Your blood pressure is high, Ella Mae—180/110."

"Why, that can't be right!" Ella Mae underscored her contradiction with another hearty laugh. "I never have high blood pressure!"

My patient's eyelids were swollen. "How much sleep did you get last night, Ella Mae?" I asked.

"Oh, I've been too busy to sleep, Doctor! I'm so pleased with all my new clothes, and I had no idea that refrigerators are so cheap! Why, I've bought four of them already, and I'm going tonight for another one."

"Whatever will you do with five new refrigerators?" Ellen asked. We both knew that Ms. Blossom lived by herself in a farmhouse that she had inherited from her parents years ago.

Ella Mae giggled mysteriously. "I'll share my secret if you promise not to tell. I'm going to open a bed-and-breakfast! People have been calling around the clock for reservations. I feel really lucky to have already found all these refrigerators." She giggled again. "Dr. Jenkins, I bet you never would have guessed that all these people want to visit me in Wolftown!"

Swimming upstream against a verbal torrent, I had to admit that my patient was right. I never would have guessed that her backwoods hamlet was about to explode into a tourist Mecca. Although all three of us were native Madisonians, Ella Mae was living in a country that was foreign to Ellen and me.

"Ella Mae!" Fighting the swirling floodwaters, I interrupted my patient's chatter. "Tell me, when did you stop your lithium?"

Ella Mae told me that two weeks ago, she had flushed her entire supply down the commode. She had never liked to take her medicine, which made her feel tired and sweaty. In a stroke of good luck, she had discovered that if she ate enough pistachio ice cream, she didn't need any lithium.

I glanced at Ellen. "Ella Mae, you're exhausted from lack of sleep. You need to be in the hospital."

Hoop earrings jangled. "I absolutely will not go to the hospital! Why, Doctor, that's complete nonsense!"

As I listened to the continuing peals of laughter, I suddenly felt an inner emptiness. Perhaps it was my new diet, or perhaps it was compassion for a lonely woman who had created a delusional world filled with friends and food and fun.

I repeated my recommendation, and once again, my patient emphatically rejected it. After only ten minutes together, we had arrived at a therapeutic impasse. The Code of Virginia clarifies the ancient issues of personal freedom and social responsibility, but in a real-life situation, the physician's arbitrating role is often uneasy and ambiguous.

I reviewed our options. In the preferred scenario, Ella Mae would choose voluntary psychiatric hospitalization, and I would arrange this. Or if she declined this approach, I could obtain a temporary detaining order mandating an involuntary trip to Staunton.

Trickles of tears melted Ms. Blossom's cosmetic mask. "Please, Doctor, don't make me go back to that awful place."

"I'm just trying to help you," I said softly.

Collapsing into Ellen's arms, my patient sobbed like a child.

The county magistrate informed me that, on this Friday afternoon, the judge had already left for his weekend retreat. Still, the temporary detention order (TDO) should be available within two hours, and a sheriff's deputy would transfer Ella Mae to Staunton. I explained the plan to Ella Mae. Her grief-stricken eyes haunted me for the rest of my afternoon.

I was finishing my dictation when I heard a sound that is unusual in a medical office. Someone was singing. Pausing outside Ella Mae's door, I listened to her mezzo-soprano voice repeating the familiar words of an old Protestant revival hymn—"Just as I Am." In her bewilderment, my patient was singing a dirge for all the joys that could have been.

"It won't be much longer," I told Ellen as I glanced at my watch.

Our patient, with hands clasped and eyes closed, sang for us. "Just as I am, poor, wretched, blind; sight, riches, healing of the mind, yea, all I need in Thee to find, O Lamb of God, I come, I come."

I tiptoed out of the room like I was departing prematurely from church. Ellen followed me, and I asked if there were any family members we should call.

"Nobody that you'll want to," she replied. My patient's only brother, Lester Blossom, had a thicker psychiatric file than his sister did and wasn't nearly as sociable. He lived in Greene County, and on one occasion, he had fired a gun at a door-to-door vacuum cleaner salesman.

"Let's not call him," I agreed. Somehow Lester didn't sound like a promising new ally.

Waiting for the TDO, I listened to scores of stanzas from "Just as I Am." As a revival-going child, I had endured many prolonged altar calls, but even for me Ella Mae's marathon broke all the records.

When Deputy Pete Harris finally arrived, he was potbellied, had a pistol in his holster, and ignored our no-smoking signs.

"So old Ms. Blossom has gone off again, has she?" Deputy Pete Harris covered Ellen's frown with a cloud of cigarette smoke. Reaching into his pocket, he pulled out a sheaf of papers. "So you're Ella Mae Blossom, Wolftown, Virginia?"

Ella Mae responded to this recitation by closing her eyes. "Just as I am, Thou wilt receive, O Lamb of God, I come, I come."

I didn't catch what Deputy Harris muttered, but it sounded irreligious. From his pocket, he produced a pair of handcuffs.

"Oh, she doesn't need those," Ellen objected.

"Sheriff's office policy, ma'am." As Deputy Harris restrained a pair of prayerful wrists, he exhaled two streams of blue smoke. "You never know when one of these loonies will try to bolt, do you, Doc?"

In an uncomfortable recessional, the four of us walked out to the shiny brown cruiser parked beside Ella Mae's dusty Plymouth. As Deputy Harris fastened his charge's seat belt, she was still singing her song. Through the twilight, my nurse and I watched the cruiser race out of the parking lot and tear down the highway.

"I don't think he needs to drive that fast," I commented.

Ellen glanced at me. "Dr. J., if you had to listen to an endless recording of 'Just as I Am,' you might feel differently. By the time those two get to Staunton, Deputy Harris will need psychiatric treatment himself."

Ellen covered her ears and laughed. "And as for me, I'll never go to another revival as long as I live!"

On my drive home, the final embers of the evening sun silhouetted the Blue Ridge Mountains. The familiar peaks looked like dark purple spikes of cardboard projecting into a coral sky.

When I rounded the final curve on County Road 631, I was ravenous. But with my family away for the week, I decided to be Spartan and to reinforce my diet with tuna and cucumbers. I was already in our driveway before I spotted the battered green pickup with the Confederate flag decal and the gun rack.

On this winter evening, the darkness had fallen quickly, and I couldn't actually see the face of the tall thin man standing beside the pickup.

"How can I help you, sir?" I asked.

My visitor's handshake was strong and callused. "So you're the doctor that saw Ella Mae." His voice was low baritone imprisoned in granite. "I'm her brother, and I want to know why you sent her to Staunton."

As I strained to see the speaker, my heart pounded. My sympathetic nervous system was kicking in with its primordial overdrive of fight-or-flight. Just now, neither option looked especially promising. "How did you know that your sister isn't well?"

Lester Blossom kicked the gravel with his work boots. "Ella Mae came by my place after midnight, and she was all worked up. Sis gets that way sometimes. I was following her around today when I saw the sheriff's car at your office." His boot traced a careful arc in the gravel. "So why did you send her to Staunton, Doc? Ella Mae's never hurt anybody."

Fifty yards away across a frozen lawn, our nearest neighbors were watching the evening news. Reflected in their living room window was the blue glare of their television. Staring through the dusk at my interrogator, I wondered if I would be part of tomorrow's headlines.

"So why did you send her to Staunton, Doc?" Lester Blossom stepped a little closer.

My voice, usually robust, was a shadow of its old self. Carefully choosing my words, I explained my worries about his sister's exhaustion and the possibility that she might hurt herself.

Lester dismissed my concerns by noting that his sister was too religious to commit suicide. Stepping backward, he leaned against his rusty fender. "Ella Mae's just a really good woman, just a really good woman, Doc." His voice was so hushed that, under the blanket of the night, I wondered if a child was crying.

"Has Ella Mae always enjoyed singing so much?" I asked

Lester looked startled. "When did you ever hear her sing?"

"Just this afternoon, Mr. Blossom. She has a beautiful voice. She must really like 'Just as I Am.'"

Lester hesitated before confiding his answer to the darkness of our front yard. "That's her favorite hymn. She and I used to sing that song as a duet when we were just kids."

"Maybe when Ella Mae is feeling better, you can both sing it again."

After a very long ten seconds, my visitor nudged the gravel. "Maybe so," he said. Then there was another callused handshake, and his truck was backing over our lawn. Only the left taillight was working, and this solitary red beacon wobbled, flickered, and finally disappeared around the bend of County Road 631.

When I unlocked our side door, my hands were shaking. "It must be really cold out here tonight," I said to myself, "or maybe it's this new diet." Pushing the door open, I flipped on the kitchen lights and fastened the safety bolt.

In the midst of life, we are in death, I reflected as I flipped back the tab on the first beer I had drunk in six months. I was relishing its cold, crisp bubbles when I discovered my wife's note on the microwave.

> *Dear, I rewired the furnace, and it's working fine. You'll find a meat loaf and two dozen fresh rolls in the refrigerator and a chocolate cake on the dining room table. Enjoy! See you Monday.*
>
> —*Doreen*

Man's days are brief upon the earth, I reminded myself as I cut off a second slab of chocolate cake. *I can always diet tomorrow. After all, a country doctor has to keep his strength up. You never know when he may need it!*

CHAPTER SIXTEEN

THE KNOCK ON THE DOOR

Not many sounds in life, and I include all urban and all rural sounds, exceed in interest a knock at the door.
—Charles Lamb, *Essays of Elia*, 1823

Rap, rap, rap! The loud knocking on the locked front door echoed through the darkened rooms of our small office. At 6:30 p.m. on this frosty February evening, our long line of patients had come and gone, and only Ellen and I were still at work.

"You'd think they could tell that we're closed," Ellen whispered. "All the lights out front are already out."

"Maybe if we're quiet, they'll get the idea and go away."

Promptly rebutting my suggestion, our after-hours visitor pounded again. Bang, bang, bang! Somehow the knocking sounded even more urgent.

"I'd better see who it is," Ellen decided. "Maybe somebody left a purse in the waiting room and needs it before tomorrow morning."

Standing in the lab, I heard the door open and caught snatches of a brief conversation. Then Ellen guided a tall middle-aged black man toward an exam room.

"Mr. Ludson is having chest pain," she remarked. "I'll check his blood pressure and EKG and have him ready for you soon."

As the exam room door closed, I walked back to my desk and stared at its shiny glass top. Suddenly, I was seething with rage. Today I had worked far too many hours already. Crushed by the onslaught of the truly sick and the worried well, I had canceled the one bright spot on my schedule—my lunchtime tennis appointment with Mark Detamore. And now, after I had survived the gauntlet, how could this complete stranger demand an after-hours evaluation?

Mindless of my fury, Ellen opened the exam room door. "Dr. Jenkins, I need you right away. He's had chest pain for the last two hours, and I don't like the looks of his EKG."

Instantly, I knew that my nurse was right. On three of the EKG leads, ST segments rode high above the baseline—a configuration dubbed in black medical humor as the "tombstone sign." Our patient was having a heart attack, an acute myocardial infarction that was strangling the muscle on the inferior aspect of his heart.

Like a magic wand, the hyperacute EKG changes transformed my hostility into concern. I grasped my patient's hand. It was big and rough.

"Ellen, call the Rescue Squad," I said, "and then get the oxygen tank and the crash cart."

My nurse ran out the door and disappeared down the hall.

"I'm sorry you're not feeling well," I said to Mr. Ludson. On this chilly evening, his muscular chest was covered with sweat—a portent of disaster.

"It started about four thirty, Doc." Mr. Ludson gritted his teeth. "I was coming back from a plumbing job—feeling as fine as usual—and all at once, it just hit me. My chest feels like it's in a vise."

Assuring my patient that oxygen and pain medication were on the way, I listened to his chest. His breathing was regular, but his heart rate was slow—only forty beats per minute.

"Are you on any regular medications, Mr. Ludson?" I asked.

My patient shook his head. Just before Christmas, he had run out of his blood pressure medication and hadn't gotten it refilled. Glancing at the chart notes, I felt apprehensive. At 90/64, my patient's blood pressure was low.

"Doc, this pain's getting really bad. I don't know. I just don't feel right."

Suddenly, under my index finger, Mr. Ludson's radial artery went limp. His mouth sagged and his work-hardened muscles relaxed. As Ellen ran into the room, we shouted simultaneously. "Code—cardiac arrest!"

In the emergency department, "Code" is the most powerful expletive that I know—far more potent than any of the more conventional four-letter words. When anyone yells "Code!" the halls vibrate with frenzy. The racing footsteps belong to a battalion of reinforcements—respiratory therapists, IV team members, EKG technicians, and extra doctors and nurses. But in Madison, on this gloomy evening, no fresh troops would rush in to shore up our fragile battle line. Ellen and I were on our own.

"You do CPR while I ventilate," I said.

Positioning her hands on Mr. Ludson's hairy chest, my nurse swung into a lifesaving rhythm. "One, two, three, four, five, breathe! One, two, three, four, five, breathe!"

Standing behind the exam table, I tilted our patient's head and extended his chin with my fingers. Already, Mr. Ludson's ebony skin was growing pale. After selecting a plastic face mask, I secured it over his nose and mouth. As the oxygen bag filled, I squeezed the precious molecules into my patient's lungs and looked at Ellen. "Did you get through to the Rescue Squad?"

"I told the dispatcher it was an emergency. She said she'd try to have a crew here in ten minutes."

"Ten minutes! We can't wait that long!"

In a code situation, ten minutes is an eternity—a narrow slit of time in which a life can either be saved or lost. Like other local medical practices, our office had no defibrillator. On those rare occasions when we needed one, we called the Rescue Squad.

"They don't know we have a code, do they?" I asked.

"No, they don't."

In my chest, panic roared in from nowhere. Often, our Rescue Squad first responders arrived in farm boots and coveralls. Certainly, no one was likely to be carrying a defibrillator. I looked down at the helpless body on our exam table. Somewhere between life and death, Mr. Ludson was in an ephemeral transition zone.

When a heart attack victim suffers a cardiac arrest, the culprit is usually ventricular fibrillation. In this lethal development, the regular contractions of heart muscle abruptly degenerate into hundreds of irregular twitches. Circulation stops, and within a few minutes, irreversible brain damage occurs. The only effective remedy is defibrillation—the sending of an electrical discharge across the chest to quell the rebellious cells and allow the return of a normal rhythm.

"I'm going to intubate him," I said. Snapping a curved blade onto the laryngoscope, I removed my patient's face mask, opened his mouth, and saw the gleaming portal of two white vocal cords. In seconds, the tube was in his trachea.

"Call the dispatcher again," I ordered. "I can handle it until you get back." As Ellen dashed out the door, I began my new rescue rhythm—fifteen and two, fifteen and two.

I glanced at my watch. As a duo, Mr. Ludson and I were four minutes into his code.

When this Wednesday had dawned, it probably had looked like a typical day for both of us with a quick breakfast followed by a drive to work while anticipating a quiet dinner at home. But a cholesterol plaque—a sequestered saboteur in Mr. Ludson's right coronary artery—had revolutionized our evening plans.

"Two minutes!" gasped Ellen, rushing back. "I told the dispatcher to expedite everything!"

"Start an IV," I ordered, counting chest compressions with my right foot. "Then we'll be ready to shoot in the medicines when the squad gets here."

Ellen was taping down the catheter when the front door burst open. Booted feet ran toward us, and then an immense orange and blue angel filled the doorway. Instead of a halo and wings, Paramedic Rob Thorson was wearing a zippered jumpsuit, but with the defibrillator swinging from his arm, he was definitely sent from heaven.

Rob slapped two adhesive pads onto Mr. Ludson's chest and flipped on the cardiac monitor. An irregular trail of electrical jerks raced across the screen.

"Ventricular fibrillation," Rob said. I nodded.

I pushed the charge button, and the defibrillator whined.

"I'm ready!" I yelled. "All clear!"

When I pushed the button, the electric shock depolarized Mr. Ludson's chest wall, and his torso jumped. The powerful volts had obeyed my command. But on the monitor, a sinister scribble persisted—the grisly autograph of Death.

This time, we had failed. We must try again.

All around us were therapeutic sounds—the whoosh of ventilations, the creaks of the exam table yielding to our compressions, and the renewed whine of the defibrillator.

"I'm ready to shock again," I announced.

As my assistants stepped aside, I jabbed the blinking button, watched Mr. Ludson's chest jump, and studied the monitor's green tracing.

"It worked!" Ellen exclaimed. Her hazel eyes were ecstatic.

And, indeed, it had worked. After a few seconds of electrical artifact, regular cardiac impulses flowed in an orderly row across the screen. Each impulse was a gift—the gift of life from the Defibrillator Angel.

With his massive but sensitive fingers, Rob confirmed that our patient had a strong carotid pulse. As I squeezed the ventilation bag, I suddenly heard a gurgle. Then my patient's hands moved.

"It's okay, Mr. Ludson," I said. With one steady movement, I pulled out his endotracheal tube. My patient coughed and cleared his throat.

"Lidocaine, 100 mg IV bolus," I ordered.

My nurse dived into the code cart for the medication that prevents further irregularities in heart rhythm.

Rob placed an oxygen mask over Mr. Ludson's face. "How are you feeling now, sir?"

Wrinkling his forehead, our patient yawned. Then like a wrestler warming up after a nap, he flexed and extended his fingers. His answer was muffled by the oxygen mask. "Okay."

"You're doing a lot better," I agreed as I watched Ellen adjust the IV infusion.

And with every passing second, I felt better myself. Somewhere out in the night, a siren was insistent. Help was on the way.

In a few minutes, Rob's EMTs were swarming all over our office. Applying new monitoring leads, they transferred Mr. Ludson to the waiting ambulance. My telephone call to the University of Virginia Emergency Department was another model of brevity—a forty-eight-year-old male with an acute inferior wall myocardial infarction had arrested in ventricular fibrillation. He had been resuscitated and was neurologically intact.

"You'll be flying out on *Pegasus*," I said. The University's Hospital was dispatching its medevac helicopter to Madison. "And now it's time to call your family."

"Dorothy should be home by now," my patient said. "Try 555-3123."

I dialed the number, and a pleasant female voice answered after two rings. "Mrs. Ludson?" I asked.

"That's me."

"I'm Dr. Jenkins," I said, "and I need to talk to you about your husband." For a fleeting moment, I reflected on how different my message would have been if the Defibrillator Angel hadn't arrived at just the right time.

"Is Jesse all right, Doctor?"

Thankful that I could offer a qualified yes, I informed Mrs. Ludson about her husband's heart attack, his cardiac arrest, and the planned transfer by *Pegasus*. Mrs. Ludson said that she would meet us at the high school parking lot, which doubled as the county helipad.

When our ambulance reached the parking lot, *Pegasus* was waiting. The helicopter's blades hurled arcs of light across the nearby football field, which was already alive with the police cruiser light bars. As I jumped down from the ambulance, a gray-haired black woman in a light blue topcoat hurried over.

"Is Jesse still doing okay, Doctor?" Mrs. Ludson asked.

I turned and looked as the EMS crew hoisted the big man and his stretcher out onto the pavement. "I think so, Mrs. Ludson, but come see for yourself."

Mrs. Ludson needed no second invitation. Sweeping past Ellen and me, she clutched her husband in her arms.

"Honey!" Her voice was so intense that it cut through all the noise from *Pegasus*. "Honey, are you all right?"

Rob loosened the stretcher straps, and Mr. Ludson leaned forward into his wife's welcome. "It's mighty good to see you, Dorothy."

Judging by her loud smacking kiss, Mrs. Ludson felt the same way.

With its usual deafening roar, the mighty flying horse lifted off into the night sky and disappeared over the poplar trees, heading for the University's coronary care unit. Standing in the parking lot, I stared into the sky until the last blinking red signal faded from sight.

For me, even after years of emergency medicine, a helicopter transfer is unfailingly dramatic. Somehow it makes me think about the Prophet Elijah's ascent to heaven in his chariot of fire.

As I walked back to the ambulance, someone touched my arm. It was the lady in the blue topcoat.

"Dr. Jenkins, in all the uproar, I forgot to ask you how Jesse got in to see you. He doesn't ever like to go to the doctor, and I didn't know that you had such late office hours."

Standing together by the football field, a raw wind blew into our faces. I thought about the after-hours knock and my initial reaction to it.

"Our office was already closed, Mrs. Ludson, but your husband knocked on the door, and we let him in."

When Mrs. Ludson looked at me, she was staring right through me like a hiker straining to see a distant mountain—a mountain almost lost in the mist. When she spoke, her voice was several decibels lower. "I'm so glad you were there for Jesse when he needed you, Doctor. I just don't know how to thank you."

When Ellen and I arrived back at the office, the post-resuscitation debris was impressive. As we sorted through needles, syringes, catheters, and tubes, my nurse broke the silence.

"Well, Dr. J., I guess from now on, whenever I hear somebody knocking, I'll have to open that door."

"I guess so," I said. "I'm certainly glad that you did this time."

CHAPTER SEVENTEEN

MRS. SIMPSON ATTACKS PORNOGRAPHY

**And many are afraid of God—
And more of Mrs. Grundy.**
—Frederick Locker-Lampson, "The Jester's Plea," 1868

"Dr. J., you're going to meet one of my neighbors this afternoon." Ellen's enigmatic half-smile immediately captured my attention.

Just recharged by my midday tennis match with Mark Detamore, I was ready to tackle anything. In our lunchtime get-togethers, the only thing more challenging than Mark's backhand serves was our wide-ranging conversations. Against the predictable chatter of our little town, they stood out like summer lightning.

"Should I be excited, Ellen?" I asked.

"Maybe. Dora Simpson isn't your typical patient. For starters, she's booked both of your last two appointment slots."

Stretching my shoulders, I felt the pleasant stiffness of muscles that have been pushed to exhaustion. "So she either has lots of medical problems or lots of money?"

Ellen said that neither of my assumptions was correct. Mrs. Simpson was a healthy woman of modest means. A lifelong housewife without any children, her husband had died unexpectedly about six months ago. Overall, she seemed to be adjusting reasonably well to her loss.

"So why is your neighbor coming in?"

"Just to check you out in case she needs something in the future. When she called last week, she said that for now, she's as healthy as a horse."

Mrs. Simpson must be an unusually cautious lady, I decided. Most Madisonians opted to meet me for free—at church, at the gas station, or at the grocery store. Mrs. Simpson was the first person who was willing to trade dollars for the privilege.

Standing outside the exam room, I scanned Ellen's nursing assessment. "Refuses weight and blood pressure. Feels fine. Just wants to meet the doctor."

"Hello, Mrs. Simpson," I said as I entered the room.

The matronly occupant of the armchair nodded in my direction. In her tan woolen suit and white blouse, Mrs. Simpson was thoroughly respectable. Around her black straw hat was an aureole of netting that covered iron gray hair—hair that was wrapped tightly around a roller. Seamed stockings were not strong enough to keep my patient's ankles from spilling over the sides of her thick-soled black shoes.

My late-afternoon optimism was flagging. I stoked its dwindling coals. "It's nice to meet you, Mrs. Simpson."

Relaxing her grip on a very large and very black pocketbook, my visitor shook my hand firmly. "Dr. Jenkins, I'm here this afternoon just to meet you. I don't have any medical problems, and as a sensible woman, I don't expect any. But in this world, you never know."

Without any cosmetics, her face bore the marks of time. "Yes, you never know," I agreed.

"So if I do need a doctor in the future," continued Mrs. Simpson, "I want to have the comfort of knowing what I'm getting into. I don't want any last-minute surprises."

My patient's hairnet bobbed the cadence of her sentences.

"You're a very careful person, Mrs. Simpson. Most people aren't so organized in planning their medical futures."

"Well, I'm not like most people." Something in her expression indicated that she had no regrets about that difference. "Most people that I know are entirely too careless in the way they choose a doctor."

I asked Mrs. Simpson if she had seen many physicians herself.

The hairnet wobbled in the negative. "Not many, I'm glad to say. But after my husband's stroke, he saw enough doctors to count for both of us."

Simple Gifts

I nodded sympathetically as Mrs. Simpson noted that she had lost track of the never-ending parade of doctors that were part of her husband's two-week hospitalization.

"Your husband's death must have been a great shock for you."

Pudgy fingers readjusted a pearl-tipped hatpin. "That's true. And one of the most shocking things was that first emergency room doctor. Why, he wore his hair in a ponytail tied with a red ribbon! He didn't look like a doctor at all!"

Intercepting her analytical look, I felt sure that my own closely cropped hair merited Mrs. Simpson's approval. My patient extracted her hatpin, frowned, and inserted it into another area of her ample headdress. She moved in quick stabs like she was impaling an unlucky burglar.

"Well, a doctor should at least look like a doctor. It's completely disgraceful how the average man dresses these days, anyhow, but a doctor should be different. He should set a moral standard for others to follow."

In an undisguised inspection, Mrs. Simpson surveyed my attire. Under my white lab coat was a pinstriped shirt, but my conservative tie had shifted to the left. With a casual flip, I corrected its subversive tendency.

The hairnet signaled its approval. "Some of Gordon's ICU doctors didn't wear ties at all. Can you imagine them coming to work in jeans and polo shirts?" Mrs. Simpson's voice was scandalized, as if she were describing a colony of hospital-based nudists.

"All in all, the University doctors were a most unsatisfactory lot," concluded my patient as she noted my scuffed oxford slippers. "And with the cost of hospital care nowadays, Heaven knows that doctors make enough money to buy ties and get decent haircuts."

Settling onto my stool, I said that the rising cost of health care was a real concern.

The hairnet lurched. "Gordon's bill was outrageous. Do you know that his hospital charges for those two weeks were higher than what we paid for our first house?"

I nodded meekly.

In triumph, my patient rolled past her rhetorical question. "It's outrageous, that's what it is! There's probably no limit to what doctors will do nowadays to get their hands on everybody else's money."

Mrs. Simpson gripped her black pocketbook as if purse snatching might have been an integral part of my medical school curriculum.

I remarked that my office charges seemed reasonable. In 1986, our brief office visit cost $15.00, and our standard visit is $20.00.

"Well, they're certainly not as low as Dr. Rucker's charges used to be."

When I thought about my professional predecessor, I tried to look neutral. Dr. Rucker had been an unmarried woman whose medical office was in her basement. Her financial overhead, unlike mine, was probably zero.

"Dr. Rucker was a very special person, wasn't she, Mrs. Simpson?"

Mrs. Simpson paused before casting a stone at Madison's own medical saint. "Dr. Rucker was all right in her own way. But I always thought she should have gone with the rest of us to church on Sundays."

My patient radiated the smug superiority of the religious establishment.

I suggested that at times a small-town doctor may not feel as excited about community events as other people do. At almost every social activity that I attended, I was pelted with medical questions—unlabeled orange pills to be identified, a diaper rash to be examined, a nebulous headache longing for an official name.

"It may be difficult," my visitor conceded, "but we still have to hold up the standard for other people to see."

Flitting through my imagination was an image of Mrs. Simpson—attired in her tan suit and hatpin—running up a banner over an ecclesiastical barricade.

My visitor squashed my fantasy. "So I'm glad to hear that you do go to church, Dr. Jenkins. Since so many of your colleagues don't nowadays, it's even more important for you to set a good example."

Uncomfortable under the weight of my exemplary behavior, I said that while I enjoyed church music, perhaps Dr. Rucker had not.

In fact, we both knew that this was the undeniable truth. Dr. Rucker had been so absorbed in her medical practice that she rarely took time for anything else. Mrs. Simpson, choosing to ignore my wishy-washiness, announced her decision to see only doctors who attended church regularly.

As a card-carrying Methodist, I smiled.

"And doctors shouldn't ever use tobacco either," she continued. Above us, her banner rippled in the breeze. "Dr. Rucker smoked all the time. Such a bad example for our youth."

In fact, Dr. Rucker had defied public opinion by chain-smoking her way through carloads of thin brown Cuban cigarettes. I said that it was too bad when someone got hooked on tobacco.

Simple Gifts

The hairnet shook its disapproval as Mrs. Simpson declared that she absolutely had no sympathy for cigarette smokers and that she held them accountable for their own moral failings.

Casting about for a response, I noted that our office was a nonsmoking facility.

"And doctors need to keep away from alcohol," continued Mrs. Simpson. Her voice was charged with the fervor of a crusading abolitionist.

Thinking about the two or three bottles of red wine reposing on our pantry shelf, I felt a sudden warmth. Did Mrs. Simpson plan to inspect the cellars and storerooms of her prospective physicians?

Mrs. Simpson noticed my flush. "Well, Dr. Jenkins, don't you agree that it's morally wrong to use alcohol?"

Sidestepping perjury, I carried the war into the enemy's country. "Are you asking me, Mrs. Simpson, whether the inappropriate use of alcohol is more medically harmful than other unwise habits, such as overeating?"

My patient made several futile downward tugs at her overstretched tan skirt and then looked at me with unmistakable coolness. Behind the barricade, she had not foreseen this wing tipped arrow aimed at her personal armor.

Reinforcing my attack, I noted that I saw far more patients whose health problems were associated with overeating than with excessive drinking. While Mrs. Simpson grudgingly allowed that this might be so, it was apparent that she considered my counterassault to be in poor taste.

Looking into her earnest scowl, I tried to remember when I had last enjoyed a glass of wine. Far too long ago, I decided. By tonight, I would have earned one. The clandestine thought cheered me considerably.

"I don't think my alcohol use will be a problem," I fudged.

Mrs. Simpson, like a priest who has just extracted a half-truth from a troublesome penitent, said that she was glad to hear it.

When she looked down at her gold watch, my optimism stirred—the end was in sight. I thanked her for coming and wished her continued good health.

Fingering her hatpin, Mrs. Simpson ignored my smile. "There's just one more subject that we need to discuss before I go."

Like a goose shot out of the sky, my hopes plummeted.

From the depths of her cavernous purse, Mrs. Simpson recovered a pair of half-lens spectacles. Putting them on, she stared at me. "In your waiting room, Doctor, I found something that really disturbs me—something that would disturb any decent woman."

Looking over at the defending guardian of feminine virtue, I saw her pick up a recent issue of *Newsweek*. Plump fingers flipped slowly through the pages. "Here it is!" she declared triumphantly. "Now just what is this doing in your waiting room?"

Leering back at us from the magazine was a muscular male model garbed only in a rather skimpy pair of briefs. I glanced at Mrs. Simpson. "I'm sorry that you find this underwear advertisement offensive."

"This is more than offensive, Doctor," Mrs. Simpson declared. "This is pornography!"

Reflecting on my historic accomplishment in opening the first porn shop in my hometown, I asked Mrs. Simpson what she thought I should do about it.

The hairnet rose in surprise. "Dr. Jenkins, it certainly isn't my responsibility to decide what your moral obligations are."

Through my late-afternoon haze, I could still recognize a logical paradox. Gingerly, I backed away from it, and Mrs. Simpson modified her stance.

"Well, at the very least, Doctor, you have to be held accountable for the literature in your waiting room."

As I looked at the hairy legs of the fashion model, I pointed out that different advertisements may attract or repel different people. If I clipped out all possible sources of irritation, there might not be much left in some magazines.

"Then you shouldn't subscribe to such trash in the first place!" Stroking her hatpin, Mrs. Simpson glowered at the *Newsweek*. "Doctor, how would you feel if your mother saw these kinds of pictures in her son's medical office?"

Somehow I was inwardly certain that this would not be a problem. Still, I decided not to say that Mom—always overworked in her orchard—would be unlikely to waste time by flipping through a stack of my magazines.

Instead, I ventured that perhaps it might be helpful if we could think about why we react so strongly to certain types of advertising. Noting that I was always riveted to pictures of expensive sports cars, I wondered what that fascination might be trying to tell me.

Mrs. Simpson's eyebrows told me that she didn't think the message would be very uplifting. "That's not the way I look at morals, Doctor."

Simple Gifts

Closing the *Newsweek,* I placed it on the exam table. "Well, Mrs. Simpson, why do you think that we humans act the way we do? Even when we don't really need sports cars, we drool over the advertisements, and at the risk of our very lives, we smoke cigarettes, drink too much alcohol, and eat too many desserts."

My visitor straightened in the armchair. "It's because most people are bad, just naturally rotten to the core. And the way I see it, it's up to the rest of us to stand up for all the right things."

Her pronouncement rang through the exam room with the clarity of a vespers bell.

"But I wonder," I hedged, "if sometimes when we go after unhealthy and unwise things, there may be another reason. Maybe, inside ourselves, we have this big black hole—an empty spot that we keep trying to fill up anyway we can."

Mrs. Simpson shrugged. "I don't know, Doctor." Standing, she repeated her doubt more slowly. "I don't know."

At the checkout counter, Ellen was waiting for us. Outside the windows, the shroud of early evening lay over the white pines. I watched as Mrs. Simpson drove away.

"There, to my mind, goes a very lonely woman," remarked Ellen. "I live two houses down from her, and I've only seen her once since her husband died."

"That's too bad."

"But you got to see her for quite a while today, didn't you?" Mischief twinkled in Ellen's hazel eyes. "So tell me now, Dr. J., did you pass muster with Dora?"

I shrugged. "I guess that Mrs. Simpson is the only one who can answer your question. After all, she does hold her physicians to rather high standards."

Ellen smiled as she clicked off her desk light. "Maybe so. But if I had to bet on it, I'd say you'll be seeing her again someday."

CHAPTER EIGHTEEN

CHOLESTEROL SCREENING AND SAUSAGE GRAVY

> **No lesson seems to be so deeply inculcated by the experience of life as that you should never trust the experts. If you believe the doctors, nothing is wholesome.**
> —Lord Salisbury, letter to Lord Lytton, June 1877

─✦─

Driving along through the fog before sunrise, I knew that I was still half-asleep. On this Sunday morning, my alarm clock had gone off at the pathologically early hour of 6:00 a.m. Soon, I would be arriving at the Rescue Squad building to assist with the Health Awareness Breakfast.

In 1986, the research results were already in. A high-fat diet was a major contributing factor to the American epidemic of coronary artery disease. As a health maintenance effort, we physicians were encouraging our patients to reduce their serum cholesterol levels to less than 240 milligrams per deciliter.

And to nurture this fledgling public health effort, the Madison Rescue Squad was sponsoring the first free cholesterol screening program in our county. Preparing for this event, I had picked up informational materials from the Heart Association office and would be on the scene to interpret lab results.

"But why do we have to start so early?" I grumped as I stopped in an almost empty parking lot. Grabbing a display poster and three boxes of Healthy Heart diet brochures, I marched up the frozen walkway.

Stepping inside, I instantly was wide-awake.

In the expansive warmth of the banquet room, the rich aromas of a hot breakfast swirled around me like an olfactory concert. There was the basso profundo of freshly brewed coffee, the tenor warmth of baking biscuits, and the spicy alto of fried apples. And above it all was the melody line—savory country sausages flavored with sage and simmering together on oversized griddles.

"Hi, Doc!" On hand to greet me was Paramedic Rob Thorson, who looked larger than ever in his blue and orange coveralls. "Let me help you with those boxes."

After we stacked the diet brochures on a nearby table, I taped the Healthy Heart poster to the wall. Rob scrutinized the Heart Association's conception of a breakfast buffet. Surrounding a prim bouquet of red and white carnations was an array of low-fat foods—whole grain breads, high-fiber cereals, fresh fruit, sundae glasses filled with peach yogurt, and a pitcher of tomato juice.

"Well, I'm glad we don't have to try to raise money by selling that stuff," he said. "We believe in real food around here."

Joining us in inspecting the peach yogurt was a young woman—fresh and efficient in an olive uniform—who introduced herself as the visiting lab technician. With professional pride, she informed me that her diagnostic analyzer could process ten cholesterol assays every two minutes. Suitably impressed, I asked if she had run any samples this morning.

The technician awarded me the special smile reserved for prospective patients. The first lab batch would include my blood sample. My eyes widened, and Rob grabbed my elbow.

"Doc and I will be back in just a few minutes," he promised. "Right now, we have to talk to Bea."

As we strolled toward the sounds of rattling pan lids, the aroma of hot food—already powerful—became almost incapacitating. Like a pilgrim kneeling on the threshold of a shrine, my stomach worshipped its new environment.

In front of us, half-a-dozen kitchen workers bustled around grills, ovens, and tables. A plump gray-haired woman with a white apron turned toward us.

Simple Gifts

"Bea, I want you to meet Dr. Jenkins," said Rob. "How long have you been cooking for us, Bea?"

"For longer than any woman would be willing to admit!" Picking up a floral print kitchen towel, Bea wiped the flour off her hands and then glanced with proprietary pride at trays filled with freshly baked biscuits.

I sniffed my appreciation. "I'm looking forward to a wonderful breakfast."

Bea's pink face broke into a wreath of hospitable wrinkles. "Well, I certainly hope that you enjoy it, Doctor. After all these years, I've never changed my recipes even once. Everybody seems to like my cooking just the way it's always been."

When Rob commented that we would return after our cholesterol checks, the cook offered me a nod that was part apology, part defiance. "Oh, I'm sure that cholesterol is important, but somehow I just like to eat what I want without always worrying about it. Why, I have a teenage granddaughter who's as skinny as a rail, and she won't eat anything made with real country butter! She's always after me to use that new-fangled low-fat stuff."

Bea wrinkled her nose—still adorned with a smudge of flour—and stared at me. Her gray eyes defended her professional heritage against the intrusions of modern medical meddlers.

Like a seasoned diplomat, Rob headed off the clash. Patting Bea's ample shoulder, he assured her that we would be right back to tackle her latest feast.

In just a few minutes, the diagnostic deed was done. The technician scrubbed my finger, and I felt a sharp jab. The machine whined, flashed, and beeped, and the printer spit out a roll of numbers.

Like an ancient Greek sibyl offering glimpses of the future, the technician handed us our results. With Rob's value at 196 and mine at 208, we were both cleared for breakfast.

Bea's cooking was everything that I had anticipated and more. With unrestrained enthusiasm, Rob and I tackled hot biscuits through which rivulets of butter flowed like subterranean streams. Bea's fried apples were a blend of Winesap wedges, nutmeg, cinnamon, and brown sugar. Crusty brown sausages popped like tiny geysers in my mouth. And the thick white gravy was a blue-ribbon example of Southern home-style cooking.

Finishing my second heaping plate, I glanced at my watch. "It's almost eight o'clock," I said as I smeared a thick layer of strawberry jam onto one final biscuit. "I need to get my table set up."

Rob impaled the last survivor of a sizable tribe of sausage links. "You're right, Doc. People will start coming anytime now."

Feeling definitely overnourished, I waddled over to my table of educational materials. Opening the boxes, I arranged the diet pamphlets into orderly rows and looked again at the low-fat breakfast poster. Somehow under the bright fluorescent light, it looked even bleaker than it had an hour ago. I was gazing skeptically at the peach yogurt when two of my patients arrived.

"Why, how nice to see you, Dr. Jenkins," Mrs. Wentworth said cordially.

Trying to take a deep breath, I discovered that my effort was futile. I was completely gorged with biscuits and gravy. Forgoing speech, I offered the Wentworths a satiated smile and a low-fat diet plan.

In their wake came an unending horde of ravenous Madisonians. Spurred on by Bea's culinary fame, entire families marched through the doorway, glanced at the yogurt poster, and hurried past it into the serving line. Borne along by the crowd were Doreen and our four children, all delighted at being taken out for a hot breakfast.

Close behind them, my buddy, Mark Detamore, grinned at me. The fashionable woman beside him was not Mrs. Detamore. Mark advised me that his wife had the flu and was home in bed. Instead, his companion this morning was Maureen Wyse. Since her son's tragic death two months before, Maureen had been seeing Mark twice a week for pastoral counseling.

Maureen looked happier this morning, I decided. Maybe she was beginning to get over it.

Behind Mark and Maureen stretched an endless army of breakfast-goers. Waving his huge arms like a traffic cop, Rob tried to divert the flow toward the lab technician, but most local citizens already had a firm grip on their medical priorities. Better to risk a heart attack sometime in the future than to yield now to imminent starvation.

Bea and Company did a land-office business.

From my solitary outpost near the door, I felt more and more like St. John the Baptist—an unheeded voice, crying out in the wilderness of modern gluttony. Unfortunately, unlike the saint, my body was stuffed with the vices that my brochures preached against.

From across the hall, Rob winked at me as he tapped on the microphone. Over a few minutes, the festive uproar subsided, and the paramedic pitched his opening line. "Folks, we certainly appreciate your coming out on this cold morning. So tell me, are you having a good time?"

A deafening eruption of cheers and whistles answered his question. After Bea and her kitchen crew appeared for a curtain call—to even more tumultuous applause—Rob reminded his feasting audience of the prevalence of heart attacks in Madison and the need for preventive medicine. And then he told them that, for the first time, a free cholesterol test was theirs for the asking.

As a chorus of voices debated his suggestion, Rob tapped his microphone.

"And this morning, Dr. Jenkins is here too," he announced, pointing toward me. "When you get your cholesterol results, you can ask the doctor any questions you may have. All for free."

From nearby tables, people gawked at me as they considered the novelty of free medical advice. A shrewd native himself, Rob had appealed to one of the most basic values of Madisonians—their frugality. Soon, a line of health maintenance converts stretched halfway across the room.

The analyzer whined, flashed, and beeped, and a ripple of excitement ran through the crowd.

"What do you know!" commented a stout gentleman, clutching a lab report in his pudgy hand. "275. Now what does that mean, Doc?"

Taking several rapid gasps, I told him that his cholesterol level was too high and advised him to lower it with a proper dietary and exercise program.

"Are you saying that I need to eat less?" The gentleman's voice was boisterous. "Doc, I enjoy good food. Why, I thought that's why you and I were both here this morning!"

Surrounded by laughter, I blushed. Suddenly, I felt like a tipsy temperance lecturer at a wine-tasting festival.

"And what about my number, Doctor?" inquired a portly lady. "It's 324. Is that too high?"

"And what about mine?" said another voice, and then another, and then another.

Suddenly, I was surrounded by a mob of people who were waving lab sheets in the air and demanding immediate professional interpretation. Our rural breakfast had turned into a riot. Breathing as deeply as I could,

I worked my way through the forest of hands. And as the early birds left, many of them picked up dietary brochures.

Finally, after what felt like several hours in the middle of a buffalo stampede, I realized that the line was slowing down. I said good-bye to Ben and Emma Hottle, our dairy farming neighbors. Both of them were delighted with their cholesterol values.

"Now I can keep on putting real cream on Ben's strawberry shortcake," commented Emma as she buttoned her topcoat. Ben shot me a grateful smile.

At the very end of the line were two other familiar faces—Wade and Eula Umstadler, the owners of my favorite local restaurant. "You've had a busy morning, Doc," Wade said.

I agreed that a lot of people had turned out. Of the three hundred dietary brochures, only a handful was left.

Picking up a diet pamphlet, Eula Umstadler leafed through it. Looking at her eternally slim figure, I suspected that her breakfast had consisted of coffee and an unbuttered biscuit.

Deflecting my envious vibrations, Miz Eula replaced the brochure. "No new information here, I'm afraid. What our people really need is a good herbal supplement to offset the bad effects of dietary fat."

Even after my one-man assault on cardiac risk factors, I still retained the good sense not to lock horns with our community's leading herbalist. "That's very interesting," I remarked.

As Mrs. Umstadler adjusted her black silk scarf, a massive blue and orange figure bounded over and slapped me on the back.

"You were great, Doc!" Rob Thorson announced to me and to the departing Umstadlers. "Just great!"

Through the closing plate glass door, I glimpsed Miz Eula's disapproving frown. I savored the frosty image.

"We fed over six hundred people!" Rob enthused. "Bea had to whip up another batch of biscuits!"

"She really is a wonderful cook," I said. Although my belt was still too tight to allow me to sit comfortably, I was too tired to stand.

Rob reported that the technician had exhausted her supply of cholesterol test kits.

"Thank goodness for that!" was the Sunday morning prayer of an exhausted public health crusader.

"Oh, you'll live to fight another day," Rob assured me. "And I need to talk to you about that. The technician can come back next month for Bea's fried chicken dinner. Could you help us out again then?"

As I glanced over my shoulder at the peach yogurt poster, I felt distinct ambivalence about my morning's performance. This low-cholesterol crusade might not be impossible, but it was going to be a hard sell—to my patients, to Rob, and most of all, to myself. But after another six weeks, I reasoned, I should be able to shed the effects of my high-fat binge and be ready for another matchup with Bea.

"Sure, Rob," I said.

My friend caressed his generous abdominal girth. "That's great, Doc! That's just great!"

"Always glad to help out," I said.

CHAPTER NINETEEN

REVEREND DETAMORE STEPS OVER THE LINE

Men are nearly always willing to believe what they wish.
—Julius Caesar, *De Bellico Gallo*

～⋙⋘～

On the following Sunday morning, when I arose at the civilized hour of 9:00 a.m., I was alone in the house. Doreen and our children were away for the weekend, visiting the Ohio grandparents.

Fortunately, I remembered that it was St. Patrick's Day. Rummaging in my bureau drawer, I located my most verdant tie and put it on.

Driving along Route 29, I noticed that Mother Nature also had slipped in a tribute to the Irish saint. A tint of green brightened the willow clumps along the Robinson River. After a downpour during the night, the swollen river was orange brown with Madison County silt.

With my first glimpse of our choir director's face, I immediately knew that something extraordinary had happened. Helen's eyes—indeed, all of her middle-aged body—was filled with the pleasure created by an unexpected small-town sensation.

"Happy St. Paddy's Day, Helen!" I said, dropping my music folder onto the tabletop.

"This certainly will be a day to remember." Helen loved playing the role of the coy informant. "But surely by now, you've heard the news?"

Shaking my head, I smiled. Helen must have a really juicy headline this time.

"And I'm certain that all the Baptists will remember it forever, even if they don't want to." Our choir director glowed as she thought about the discomfiture of our co-religionists. "Nothing even close to this has ever happened in Madison since I was born."

"All right, all right!" I flipped through my folder to locate today's anthem. "So spit it out. What's the Baptist bombshell?"

"It really *is* a bombshell." Helen resented my lack of respect.

With all the deference that I could muster, I waited.

"The Baptist preacher has run off to Georgia with another woman!" Helen's voice was ecstatic. "That Mark Detamore—the one everybody talks about all the time—has left his wife and eloped with Maureen Wyse!"

In complete disbelief, I stared at Helen. Delighted with my reaction, she launched into all the scintillating details.

Reverend Detamore had left town on Wednesday, ostensibly to attend a Baptist ministers' conference in Atlanta. Keeping his wife and two teenage sons completely in the dark, he had emptied his clothes closet and his bank account and had connected with Maureen Wyse at her elaborate beachfront home on St. Simon's Island. Just last night, he had called his wife and his head deacon to tell them that he wasn't coming back.

In my hands, the anthem book lay unopened as Helen went on.

"So when all those holier-than-thou Baptists get to Deep Run Church this morning, they'll find that their prized bird has flown his coop. Oh, how I wish I could be a fly on the wall to just see all their faces."

"Why, that's a horrible thing to say, Helen! Just think how bad you would feel if you were in their shoes!"

Helen defended her Christian charity by opining that Baptists in general were sexually repressed and that a popping-good scandal might be just what the Deep Run folks needed to drag them out of the nineteenth century.

Just then, the music room door flew open, and several more choir members rushed in, all talking at once. In the ensuing hubbub, our planned rehearsal never made it off the ground.

And perhaps this was just as well. From the organist's bench, I could tell that no one in the congregation heard more than two notes of the anthem anyway. The smiles and whispers in the pews indicated that, for once, our churchgoers were enjoying a truly stimulating Sunday morning.

Simple Gifts

When our minister began his discourse on current federal legislation concerning hunger relief in the Third World, I was grateful for a quiet space to sort out some of the muddle inside my head. Reverend Weebley's background droning offered a perfect respite.

Staring down at organ keyboard, I was glad that the black-and-white pattern looked so familiar. Just now, nothing else felt the same. An earthquake had struck my hometown, and I was still coping with the aftershocks.

Yesterday afternoon, I would have ridiculed the suggestion that Mark would be anywhere this morning except in his home pulpit. Over the past few months, Mark and I had become close friends. In spite of (or, I wondered, *Could it have been because of?*) his phenobarbital tablets, Mark was the most dedicated and effective minister I had ever met.

How could such a man just walk out on his loyal parishioners at the Deep Run Baptist Church? Mark's entire congregation idolized him. No one of his caliber had ever come their way before. From his comments during our regular tennis games, he sounded happy enough with his job. Of course, he was hoping for a raise in June, and he was confident that the annual business meeting would give it to him.

And poor Mrs. Detamore and their sons! Whenever I had been around them, they had been friendly and optimistic. How were they feeling this morning? Mark had often told me about the time when his own father had vanished and about the shame and confusion that he had felt at the time. What could my friend have been thinking about?

Lost in thought when the choir stood for the benediction, I was startled. I had totally blocked out Reverend Weebley's latest political homily. Flipping through my music, I found the right page and played the chords by reflex. None of them ever touched my rattled consciousness.

In the narthex, Reverend Weebley offered his cold-fish handshake to his departing parishioners. When several silver-haired ladies chirped that today's sermon was his best ever, the reverend's pasty face colored slightly. Since I had not heard a word that he said, I just mumbled my good-bye.

In the churchyard, the chairman of the church's board of trustees was talking earnestly to the treasurer. He, at least, wasn't critiquing the sermon. Instead, he was saying how thankful he was that such a disgraceful spectacle hadn't happened in our church. Nodding her agreement, the treasurer said that she felt sorry for the Deep Run Finance Committee. A scandal like this one would be sure to blow their budget sky-high.

"Thank God that Reverend Weebley isn't that type of person," the board chairman concluded.

I was in my truck and five miles away before I realized how idiotic his last remark had been. Of course, Reverend Weebley would never run off with a wealthy socialite. He would never be able to pull it off. Every worthwhile sin requires at least a modicum of imagination. And besides, even if our minister tried to run away, Mrs. Weebley would be sure to catch him and skin him alive.

Arriving at our solitary house, I stayed just long enough to hang up my suit and tuck my St. Patrick's Day tie back into its drawer, ready for another year. Pulling on my hiking boots and parka, I headed back out to my truck. For the first time in my life, I skipped Sunday dinner, and in twenty minutes, I was hiking solo on the White Oak Canyon Trail.

On this overcast afternoon, I had the trail to myself. Marching along in a light drizzle, I thought about this St. Patrick's Day. So far, nothing had made any sense at all.

How could a gifted minister like Mark Detamore leave Deep Run Church in such a devilish mess? In his tenure of less than a year, Mark had been a powerhouse both in and out of the pulpit. Now, in this unforeseen turmoil, lots of his new members would drift quietly away, and lots of his established ones would wish that they could. If the Deep Run folks ever recovered from their minister's folly, it would take them years. And the chances were good that they would never get over it.

And how could a conscientious father abandon his family? How would Mrs. Detamore cope with the financial and emotional fallout from the weekend's unexpected explosion? Certainly, if she had any sense, she would rent a moving van and escape from the Deep Run parsonage as soon as she could. But where would she go? And how would she deal with her sons? And how would they deal with her, and with each other, and with themselves?

Another explosion—one just a few yards away in a tangle of mountain laurel—stopped me in my tracks. With a sudden and alarming roar, a covey of grouse launched itself out of the thicket to disappear into a hemlock grove. Staring after the birds, I took a deep breath.

And who is going to play tennis with me tomorrow? As unexpected as the departing grouse, this question detonated inside my head.

Ever since Mark and I had played our first game and had shared our first talk, our get-togethers had been special occasions. In my hometown,

I knew almost everybody, and almost everybody knew me. But Mark was different. Other than Doreen, he was my only real confidant, and now he was gone.

During our frequent outings, we had bounced around almost as many topics as we had tennis balls. We had talked about our backgrounds, our occupations, our hopes, and our fears. We had laughed together over our own mistakes and over the foibles and idiosyncrasies of the parishioners and patients for whom we were responsible and about the invisible ever-changing boundaries that separated us from them.

And now one of us had crossed that boundary, and his life—and the lives of many other people—would never again be the same. Thinking about Maureen Wyse, I remembered that fateful first hug from the Baptist minister, by her only son's coffin, in a small-town cemetery, surrounded by hordes of people. *Was that when Mark had stepped across some unmarked line?*

Or was it in one of their frequent counseling sessions either in his church study or in her luxurious home? Or was it on some other occasion altogether when one person was lonely and the other was vulnerable?

After a four-hour hike, I was sitting in my mother's kitchen with my socks and parka drying by the crackling fire in her woodstove. Her homemade cookies—with green icing for St. Patrick's Day—were as tasty as ever, and the mug of tea was perfect after a walk in the rain.

Mom ran her calloused fingers over my socks. "They should be dry enough to wear in a little bit. Really, Harold, a man of your age ought to know better than to walk around with wet feet."

I said that somehow I had just needed to get out for a walk.

"You're upset about that no-good Reverend Detamore, aren't you?"

There was never anything to be gained by trying to sneak around my mother. Her intuition was foolproof.

"Of course, Harold, in the first place, you need to be more careful when you're picking your friends. That scoundrel ought to have been run out of town on a rail."

I chewed my cookie deliberately as Mom went on.

"Although I expect that soon enough, he'll wish he'd never hooked himself up with that Wyse woman. You would have to be a brave man to marry that type of widow."

I swallowed my cookie. "That type of widow?"

"Well, you do know that Colonel Wyse didn't die a natural death, don't you?"

I told Mom the truth. All I knew was that he had died at home about a year after his plane crash.

"Yes, that's exactly right. After the accident, he was paralyzed from the neck down and was in one of those battery-powered wheelchairs. He was terribly depressed. Who wouldn't be? And so, of course, the sheriff's office called his drowning a suicide, and everybody felt so sorry for poor little Maureen."

Staring at my mother, I waited.

"And of course, the maid was gone when it happened. Maureen had sent her to Charlottesville to pick up something, and when she got back home at midnight, it was all over. Colonel Wyse had drowned himself in the river, and they had already recovered the body."

In silence, I sipped on my tea.

"But it never has made any sense to me—or to a lot of other people—how a paralyzed man could get his wheelchair down those front steps and across that long pasture field and into the river without Maureen ever noticing it. You'd think that even our sheriff would have figured that one out."

"But, Mom, surely you don't think that Maureen could murder someone in cold blood and get away with it?"

My mother looked at me with a mixture of scorn and patience. "Maureen Wyse is young, beautiful, and rich and used to getting whatever she wants. And as for our county law enforcement, why I could have drowned my husband a dozen times before that sheriff smelled a rat."

The certainty in my mother's voice was unsettling. Somehow it sounded like the idea of spousal homicide might have crossed her mind before.

"But most of us don't go around murdering people or doing other stupid things," she continued, handing me my toasty warm socks. "So you just be sure that you behave yourself until Doreen gets back home."

While I slipped on my socks, Mom filled a lunch bag with cookies. "Now, I mean that, Harold, you listen to me. Here in Madison, we don't need any more professional men making fools of themselves."

"Yes, Mom. I'm sure you're right about that. I'll be good."

Alone in the rain, it was a long drive home.

CHAPTER TWENTY

MRS. MIDDLEBROOK'S REVOLVER

All professions are conspiracies against the laity.
—George Bernard Shaw, *The Doctor's Dilemma*, 1911

Winter may finally be over, I thought as I walked out the back door of our office. Blowing gently through the third week in March had come a hint of seasonal magic—the first warm breezes of a Southern spring. Today it was pleasant to get outside even if I was only going on yet another house call crammed into my lunch break.

Just this morning, Mrs. Myrtle Middlebrook's name had sprouted up like a noxious weed in my daily schedule. This octogenarian had a stubborn foot infection and was making weekly trips to a Charlottesville surgeon. To save time, her family had decided to have me change her Unna's boot, a medicated plaster dressing that speeds skin healing in patients with circulatory problems.

"But why does she need a house call?" I protested.

Ellen smiled at my peevish affront to her omniscience. "Because her niece, Beth, told me that Dr. Rucker always came out to the house to see Mrs. Middlebrook."

While I nursed black thoughts about my professional predecessor, my nurse continued her defense. "Beth says that Mrs. Middlebrook is getting a little confused and that the trips to Charlottesville really upset her. She

Simple Gifts

only lives two miles down the road. Why, on a nice day like today, you'll enjoy the ride. You may catch spring fever and never come back!"

I just might, I decided, as I pulled into the driveway of a stately brick home far back from the bustle of Route 29. Parking beside a lawn shaded by graceful holly and magnolia trees, I spotted a flagstone walkway. It led toward the white columns of a front porch.

What an idyllic spot, I thought as I walked by an overgrown bayberry hedge. Just in front of me, a pair of robins fluttered into the blossoming cascade of forsythia that grew against the weathered facade of the house.

Suddenly, the front door opened, and a tall middle-aged woman ran down the steps. In her arms, she clutched a glistening Siamese cat.

"I'm so terribly sorry, Doctor," my hostess apologized. "I'm Beth, Mrs. Middlebrook's niece, and the most awful thing has happened. Not five minutes ago, a car struck my aunt's cat. I heard Olivia yowling, and I think she has a broken leg. What do you think?"

As a physician, I usually do not venture opinions on feline orthopedic problems, but I could tell from the unnatural angulation of Olivia's left front paw that Beth was right. I nodded.

"I've already called our veterinarian," Beth informed me as she hurried down the walk. "I'll be back as soon as I can."

Glancing first at my watch and then at the rapidly retreating figure, I called after her. "Shall I go ahead and check on your aunt? Or should I wait for you to come back?"

Beth had already reached the white Lincoln Town Car before she telegraphed her reply. "Go ahead, Doctor. Front door's unlocked. Aunt Myrtle's in her bedroom. I'll be back soon!"

I watched as the Lincoln kicked up a shower of loose gravel and shot out of the driveway. Gripping my medical bag, I climbed the steps and crossed the gray-painted boards of the front porch. Lifting the antique doorknocker, I let it fall loudly against the brass plate. From inside the house, there was no answer.

I knocked twice more before I gave up. Glancing at my watch, I pushed open the front door and stepped into a wainscoted foyer, where faded floral print wallpaper hung above cherry paneling. The musty staleness of an airless house met me just inside the door.

"Mrs. Middlebrook!" I called. "I'm here to see you."

Simple Gifts

Glancing up a flight of steps, I wondered if my patient's bedroom was upstairs or downstairs. Ticking contentedly, a grandfather clock offered no suggestions.

"Mrs. Middlebrook!" I shouted, stepping onto a dingy oriental carpet in a large adjoining living room. "Where are you?"

There was no answer.

Well, Aunt Myrtle isn't likely to be in here, I decided, as I glanced at a dusty but magnificent grand piano. Its mahogany legs rested on bronze lion paws, and the yellowed keys were genuine ivory.

Maybe she's deaf and can't hear me, I thought. Venturing cautiously down a shadowy hall, I passed under the solemn surveillance of Robert E. Lee and Stonewall Jackson, who gazed down at me from larger-than-life portraits.

"Mrs. Middlebrook!" I tried again. "Where are you?"

From behind a closed door to my left, something rustled. After a moment's hesitation, I knocked loudly, turned a cut-glass doorknob, and pushed the door open. Pungent sickroom smells—the combined odors of an airless house, soiled bandages, and stale urine—hit me like an unexpected slap.

I forgot all about the stench when I saw the gun. Sitting in front of me on a canopied four-poster bed was a thin woman whose scanty white hair seemed to point in all directions at once. She was holding an oversized wooden-handled pistol, and she was pointing it directly at me.

"Stay right where you are!" ordered my newest patient in a high-pitched quaver. Her injunction was completely unnecessary. I was rooted to the spot.

"And what are you doing in my house?" demanded Mrs. Middlebrook, glaring at me through gold-rimmed spectacles. Her pistol was at least eighteen inches long and was uncomfortably close to my chest. Under my oxford shirt, I felt the clamminess of a cold sweat.

"I'm Dr. Jenkins," I said in what I hoped was a reassuring tone. "You're Mrs. Myrtle Middlebrook, and your niece, Beth, asked me to check your foot."

"You're no doctor of mine," declared Mrs. Middlebrook, gripping her weapon with renewed vigor. "Why, I've never seen you before! I don't know who are, mister, but I'm sure about one thing—you're not Dr. Rucker."

As I glanced at the commode chair and the aluminum walker, I offered a weak smile. "Why, you're right, Mrs. Middlebrook," I croaked. "But Dr. Rucker has moved away, and I'm the new doctor."

Looking at the imposter in her bedroom, Mrs. Middlebrook's skepticism was unappeased. "So where is Beth now?" Under the weight of the antique firearm, her blue-veined hands were shaking.

Inside my chest, something began to pound in an alarming fashion. *Now just stay calm*, I told myself as I thought about how hostages survive. *Just keep talking.*

"Oh, I thought you knew, Mrs. Middlebrook," I replied matter-of-factly. "Beth has taken your cat to the veterinarian's office. She'll be right back."

Looking at the ominous black hole at the end of her gun, I thought about the two Confederate generals outside in the hall. What strategy would they recommend for my predicament? Should I bolt from the room, hoping that my enemy would prove to be a poor shot? Or should I rush forward in a preemptive strike and try to knock her gun away?

My patient's torso steadied with a new resolve. "That does it. There's nothing wrong with my cat. Olivia ate her entire saucer of creamed tuna fish for lunch just like she always does."

"I'm sure you're right, Mrs. Middlebrook." I suppressed an irrational surge of hatred for her hearty house pet. "Olivia isn't actually sick, but she was struck by a car this afternoon. I saw her broken leg just as Beth left for the veterinarian's office."

Looking into watery blue eyes, I pressed my case. "I'm here to help you, Mrs. Middlebrook. Beth tells me that you've had a lot of trouble getting your foot to heal."

Mrs. Middlebrook gave a quick downward glance to her pink bedroom slippers. "I've been keeping my foot wrapped, but I don't think it's helping very much."

"And that's why I'm here, Mrs. Middlebrook, to change your bandage."

Wrinkling her forehead, my patient looked doubtful. "Beth didn't tell me that a new doctor was coming. I heard shouts in my living room and thought you were a burglar."

Through the faded lace curtains and the closed Venetian blinds floated a welcome sound—the crunching of gravel on the driveway. Hope surged into my arteries, competing with a supersaturated level of adrenaline.

"Mrs. Middlebrook, this must be your niece now. Beth can explain everything as soon as she gets here."

The front door slammed, and a pair of shoes clattered down the hallway. "Oh, Dr. Jenkins, I'm so relieved! Olivia is going to be okay. I'm sorry that I had to run out on you like that."

Simple Gifts

Beth's face was sweaty. Suddenly, her apologetic expression changed to shock.

"Aunt Myrtle!" she exclaimed, snatching the gun from my patient's hands. "What on earth are you trying to do?"

"She thought I was a burglar," I said as I took a breath.

Even in the stagnant sickroom, it felt incredibly good to breathe. I took several more deep breaths, as if I were practicing a newly acquired artistic skill. They all felt fine. It also felt good to see the antique handgun lying idle on the dressing table.

"But where could Aunt Myrtle have gotten a gun?" Beth's confusion was evident. "I'm here every day, and I've never seen any gun before."

With a kindly smile, my patient explained that she had kept a loaded pistol in her bedside table ever since her husband's death thirty years before. This precaution seemed to help her sleep better.

"In this day and time, we old people have to be able to protect ourselves," concluded Mrs. Middlebrook. Her tone was prudent, conciliatory, almost apologetic. "As long as I have my gun, nobody's going to ransack this house until they deal with me first."

"You can say that again," I agreed as I continued to savor the delights of respiration. "So now let's take a look at your foot."

Beth helped me loosen her aunt's thick cotton stocking. Cutting through the plaster Unna's boot, I looked at fragile almost translucent skin.

"So here's the ulcer," I said. "They're always slow to get well on the heel."

"They must be," commented Beth, looking over my shoulder at the raw gray area that measured two by three centimeters. "Aunt Myrtle has been having dressing changes for over six weeks now."

I predicted that another six weeks would pass before the ulcer resolved. After cleaning my patient's foot with peroxide, I applied antibiotic ointment and a nonadhesive bandage. As I molded the wet plaster loops over Mrs. Middlebrook's calf, I felt her wasted muscles.

"This boot needs to stay on until next Wednesday," I said, "and then it will be time for another dressing change."

Beth's eyes filled with embarrassment. "Dr. Jenkins, it certainly would be nice if you could do Aunt Myrtle's dressing changes. But after today, I suppose that you may never want to come here again."

Gathering up my bandage scissors, I glanced at the elderly woman who was dwarfed by her canopy bed. As Beth and I talked, Mrs. Middlebrook toyed contentedly with a diamond ring that was far too large for her bony finger.

"Oh, I'm willing to come back," I said, fastening the snaps on my medical bag. "Your aunt isn't far from my office, and I can just run out here every Wednesday at lunchtime. Of course, you will need to get that gun away from her. She might really hurt somebody one of these days."

Beth pledged to have Aunt Myrtle completely disarmed within the hour.

Back in my truck, I mashed on the accelerator and covered the two miles in record time. Braking abruptly for our office turning lane, I screeched past the other cars, ran up the back walk, and burst into the office lab.

"Why, hello, Dr. J.!" Ellen greeted me. "You're running a little late, aren't you? You must have caught the spring fever. For a while there, I was wondering if you were going to come back at all."

Struggling to push my arms through the starched sleeves of a lab coat, I nodded. "For a moment, I was wondering the same thing myself."

CHAPTER TWENTY-ONE

A MAN'S TEARS

Are all men in disguise except those crying?
—Dannie Abse, "Encounter at a greyhound bus station," 1986

"Dr. J., is it okay to tack on a late appointment this evening?" Ellen's voice was hesitant. After a fast-paced day, it was already five fifteen, and she knew how enthusiastic I would be about staying late.

"Who is it this time?"

"One of your cousins, he says."

Simply because no other physicians were available, I often cared for my hometown relatives. "Which cousin, Ellen?"

"Rod Jenkins. He just got home from his construction job and wants to see you."

So it's Rod, I thought. Just this week, my mother had called to brief me about my cousin's marital troubles. After a series of skirmishes, his wife had moved out, taking their four-year-old son with her. I'd better see this one, I decided.

Ellen wrote the new name on our six o'clock slot.

An hour later, picking up the last chart of the day, I read her nursing note. "Needs sleeping pills."

I flashed back to our last family reunion. I remembered a suntanned man who roared with laughter when he spiked the volleyball.

Simple Gifts

"Hello, Rod," I said, returning a muscular handshake.

The sun and wind of multiple construction sites had textured my patient's handsomely rugged face. His bushy brown hair was so sunburned that it matched the leather of his work boots. In faded denim jeans and a corduroy shirt, Rod was an image of hearty good health—the type of patient rarely seen in medical offices.

"Sorry to keep you so late in your office, Harold." My cousin's voice was deep and resonant.

I assured him that I was accustomed to working long hours.

In the armchair, Rod's trim torso still bore the imprint of his Air Force years.

"Harold, I know that many people are glad you're here, and right now, I'm one of them."

I said that I was sorry that things weren't going well.

"I guess I need some sleeping pills." As Rod looked down at his boots, a flush deepened his tan. "I just haven't been able to sleep since Jean left. You've probably already heard all about our mess."

Looking at the dark rings under Rod's eyes, I nodded. "This must be a very hard time for you."

"Well, it's rough enough." Taking off his wristwatch, my patient methodically stretched and released its flexible band.

"So how did all of this actually start?" I reflected on my mother's colorful version of several nights before.

"It's a long story, but I guess most marriage problems fall into that category." Then in a brief statement filled with facts, Rod described for me the history of his relationship with Jean.

When Rod—fresh out of high school—had arrived in New Jersey, Jean had been a civilian secretary at the Air Force base. She had been friendly, and Rod had been lonely, and six months later, they were married. During Rod's Air Force years, their relationship had worked out well.

"Jean never wanted to move to Virginia," Rod confided to his left boot. "And that's when she really started to drink a lot." When Rod had first met Jean, she enjoyed her after-work martinis, and he enjoyed her sociability. It took three years for him to discover that she drank at other times too—sometimes during her lunch break and rather often at bedtime.

"Jean's father was an alcoholic," Rod explained, "and she often talked about the awful things he did when she was a child. For a while, I just couldn't believe that she would repeat the same crazy mistake."

I nodded. As a physician, I am amazed by the prevalence of alcohol abuse in several generations of a single family. Even in our paradoxical world, this self-destructive pattern seems inexplicable.

"Did Jean think she had a problem?"

"Not really." My patient wrinkled his forehead as he recalled that Jean always felt better when she was drinking. During moody spells, booze brightened her up.

Before moving back to his hometown, Rod had hoped that a rural setting would help his high-strung wife to relax. Actually, it seemed to have the opposite effect. Jean breezed through several part-time clerical jobs before settling into the life of an unemployed housewife. Often, when Rod arrived home in the evening, he found his wife in curlers and a housecoat, asleep on the sofa.

When Jean discovered that she was pregnant, both she and Rod were elated. They always had looked forward to being parents. Jean worked hard to control her drinking, and Rod was buoyant.

"And how did that turn out?" My question was rhetorical. We both already knew the answer.

"Well, Timmy has always been just wonderful, but even he couldn't fix everything that was broken in our marriage." Suddenly, my cousin's voice was husky. "But I'm sure the little fellow has given it his best try."

"You must really miss him." Thinking about my own first son, I remembered sleds, wagons, and piggyback rides, all touched by the wonder of a little boy.

In my patient's eyes, something glistened.

"Rod," I said softly, "you've done a good job of telling me the facts about your years as a family man. But now it's okay to tell me how you feel about it all."

A thin trickle weaved its irregular way down a tanned cheek.

"Rod, tell me about it, if you want to," I repeated.

Like a seasonal mountain stream, Rod's tears catapulted from a dribble to a torrent. Through the sobs, his words were muffled. "I never thought she'd actually leave me."

I reached over and touched a sweaty corduroy shirt. "It's going to be okay," I whispered to the little boy hidden inside a grown-up facade. "It's going to be okay."

Outside on Route 29, convoys of noisy tractor-trailers rolled by, but in the secular cloister of our exam room, the only sounds were those of a man discovering his own grief. Through the white slats of the shutters, I glimpsed red maple blossoms, swaying in the evening breeze.

Like a summer storm subsiding, sobs faded into whimpers. "I'm sorry, Harold," my patient said.

"There's nothing to feel sorry about, Rod. It's good for people to share their feelings."

Below puffy eyes, Rod's cheeks were wet. "I'm really sorry about acting this way, Harold. I guess I'm just not getting enough sleep."

Looking down at his folder, I reviewed Ellen's recommendation. "Needs sleeping pills." Then I glanced at the flowering maple tree and put the chart on the floor.

"You know, Rod, I think that there's more to all this than just your lack of sleep. Somehow I think it's really hard for us men to just let ourselves go and feel all the things that come our way—the good and the bad."

I paused, troubled by my own banality. "But even though it's really hard, I think that it's essential for us to discover our feelings and to share them with a few other people."

In the evening breeze, a maple limb tapped at the window, like a hesitant traveler hoping for sanctuary.

"I never tell anybody except Jean how I feel." Rod had regained his composure. "I just thought that's the way it's supposed to be."

"Certainly, that's the way you and I were brought up," I agreed, thinking about our childhood on rural Southern farms, where boys were trained early to keep their chins up and to never show their feelings. In both subtle and blatant ways, we were taught to behave like real boys should.

Suddenly, I thought of another afternoon when my cousin and I had been together. "Rod, do you remember when Grandmama died?"

My cousin looked surprised. "Yeah, I remember that. It's been awhile now."

In a refreshing memory, I saw again the little white-haired woman who welcomed her grandchildren by slipping on a checkered apron and whipping up batches of sugar cookies. Whenever I walked off the school bus at her house, I wound up in the kitchen, eating cookies and telling her about the ups and downs of my day.

I was away in college when the doctors diagnosed her pancreatic cancer and allotted her another six months. With native toughness, Grandmama doubled their projection, but in her final spring, she didn't plant her onions, and in August, she was gone.

Simple Gifts

"Grandmama was a very special person," Rod said.

"She certainly was." I remembered the sweltering heat at her funeral. First, we had gone to the Methodist church and then to the cemetery and finally back to Grandmama's house. "What a crowd of people were at that funeral."

Although they were still red, Rod's eyes twinkled. "We come from a big family, Harold."

"And at Grandmama's house on that afternoon," I persisted, "all the women were in one place, and all the men were in another. And both groups acted as if they were on two different planets."

Rod looked thoughtful.

"My mother and your mother were outside," I said, "walking in Grandmama's herb garden. And around the kitchen table, Aunt Lillian and Aunt Pearl were leafing through that old cookbook, reading the notes that Grandmama had written beside her recipes. First, they laughed, and then they cried. Aunt Pearl said that nobody would ever be able to make piecrust like Grandmama."

"Nobody ever will," my cousin agreed.

"And meanwhile, all the men were out on the front porch. They were dressed in their Sunday suits and were talking about how much their crops needed a good rain. I'm willing to bet you that, all that afternoon, not one of those men even mentioned Grandmama."

"That was just their way of handling it, I expect."

"But maybe it's not the best way," I objected, "for them or for anyone else. Maybe there were times when they really needed to open up, and they were just afraid."

My cousin gave me a hard look. "So have you ever taken your own advice, Doctor?"

My mind flew back to the last three months of my medical residency and to the most serious depression of my life. After slaving through seven years of postgraduate work, I soon would have to stop studying and start the actual business of living. In that April, the upcoming change hit me with the force of a freight train.

Looking out at the maple blossoms, I felt it all again.

At first, there had been the complete inability to sleep even when I had a night off. Then there was the panic attack. Driving along on the expressway, I suddenly wasn't sure where I was or even if I was anywhere. When I finally got home, I sat up all night, trying to convince myself that

I wasn't losing my mind. And as soon as the medical offices opened the next morning, I called my first psychiatrist.

On the telephone, Dr. Davidson had told me to come right in, and, fighting my phobia of psychiatrists, I had done just that. As I had walked through his door, I anticipated that he would listen to me, confirm my diagnosis of insanity, and quickly consign me to an institution.

I had not foreseen his kind eyes and his soft voice. I had also not in my wildest dreams imagined that he would touch my shoulder and tell me that I was okay or that I would sit in front of this unknown man and sob my heart out.

Perhaps we never forget what someone says to us when we are crying.

"Crying isn't for sissies," Dr. Davidson had said. "Only a strong man can be honest about his own fears."

Seven springtimes past, his words had swaddled me in their comfort, and now I was sharing them with someone else.

"Under our skins, Rod," I replied, "I expect that most men are a lot alike—all locked up inside ourselves. But eventually, if we're lucky, someone shows us a key, and then—when we're ready—we begin to unlock a series of doors."

"That could very well be the way it is, Harold. But I still think that what I need most is a long night's sleep."

Agreeing that Rod needed several of them, I prescribed a few sleeping pills, talked about maintaining rhythms in daily activities, and asked him to call me tomorrow.

Driving home, I was lost in an evening meditation about Rod and about men in general.

Why, after just losing his wife and son, was it so embarrassing for Rod to cry? Why had my father, desperate in his own bitterness, never dared to unlock the door? How could Mark Detamore have walked away from a friendship that we both enjoyed without ever saying good-bye? Six weeks had passed since that fateful St. Patrick's Day, and I had never heard a sound from my Baptist buddy.

How carefully—with what infinite care—have we males been conditioned to build our own dungeons and to hide inside their walls. How desperately—with what heart-pounding desperation—do we dread the consequences of unlocking the door.

My God, I wondered, mingling prayer with imprecation, *will we men ever, ever be able to touch each other?*

All around me, twilight veiled the hills and pastures of Madison County. On the crest of the Blue Ridge, the last glow of the departing sun touched the mountains like a benediction, like the fading notes of an evensong.

CHAPTER TWENTY-TWO

DARK SECRET ON MAIN STREET

Each has his past shut in him like the leaves of a book known to him by heart; and his friends could only read the title.
—Virginia Woolf, *Jacob's Room*, 1922

※

"What a great day to be alive!"

Driving up Madison's Main Street on my way to the office, I was a prodigal son who felt sentimental about his homecoming. All around me were the landmarks of my childhood. Unchanged by the passage of thirty years were the brick courthouse, the white clapboard houses, and the colonial Methodist Church with its graceful steeple. Even the trees—magnolia, holly, and maple—were old friends who had simply grown taller and bigger.

When I walked into my office, I was still counting my blessings. In my hyper-mobile generation, few people experience the stabilizing rhythms of growing up and growing old in the same community. Even rarer is the doctor who opens a medical practice in his hometown. For me, after nine months in my new office, the thrill still tasted as fresh as a new strawberry. After twenty years of exile, what could be finer than being back on Main Street?

"Here's a familiar name from high school days," I remarked to Ellen as I scanned the afternoon appointment book. "Becky Bentham was in my graduating class. What's she coming in for?"

Ellen shrugged. "I don't know. She needs you to refill a prescription."

"Didn't she ever get married?" Becky's surname was unchanged from our school days. "Or has she gotten divorced and taken her old name back?"

As a one-person reference text on her fellow citizens, Ellen enjoyed my curiosity. "For starters, your old school chum never met Mr. Wonderful. She's had the same job since your class graduated. She's an insurance adjuster in Charlottesville."

"Surely, she doesn't still live on Main Street?" In Madison County, while most people aren't given to change, they aren't completely immobile.

During our school years, Becky had lived with her mother and stepfather in one of the large Victorian homes on Main Street. Their house had three chimneys and dozens of green shutters that matched the tin roof. From the school bus, I often admired the wraparound porch covered with purple wisteria blossoms.

"Actually, she does," Ellen replied "Of course, she lives by herself now. You probably heard about her parents' car accident last year. Her stepfather pulled out in front of a gravel truck, and they both were killed instantly."

"That's too bad," I sympathized, thinking about the Becky of years gone by. Small-town spinsterhood was not the future that I had envisioned for the pretty teenager walking under the rose arches at graduation. But, not being a very astute seer, neither had I foreseen my own return to Madison as a medical doctor.

"Well, hello, Becky!" I said, walking into the exam room. A pleasant still- shapely woman arose from the armchair to shake my hand. My patient had acquired a few extra pounds, and her dark wavy hair was streaked with gray. But the shy smile told me that, without a doubt, I was once again talking to Becky Bentham.

An initial medical visit involving two high school friends, when rated for efficiency, does not earn a high score. As in other similar reunions, I found myself laughing about old times—about Miss Hareton's English essay questions, about Mr. McPhipps's pop quizzes, and about the basketball team for which Becky had been a star.

Lost in happy recollections, I suddenly felt the sharp jab of duty. Becky had made an appointment to see me not as an old friend but as her new physician. I stopped talking, smiled, and waited.

"I came to see you because I need my Prozac refilled," Becky announced. Trying to squelch an uneasy inner vibration, I nodded. "Since my parents died, I've been seeing a psychologist, and she gets my family doctor to prescribe my medicine. Prozac has been a big help since I started it six months ago."

I thought back to lazy afternoons at the local drugstore when a teenage basketball player had giggled over root beer floats. I said that I was sorry about her parents' accident.

"I'm still adjusting to being alone. Everything happened so suddenly that sometimes it still doesn't seem quite real." A faraway expression drifted through her gray eyes. "But Dr. Lightfoot, who's my psychologist, says that's only to be expected."

I commended my patient for seeing a professional counselor. In my experience, the combination of psychotherapy and medication usually is the most effective approach to a variety of emotional problems. Prozac was Becky's only prescription medication, and other than her depression, she generally enjoyed good health.

"I'll drop Dr. Lightfoot a note about your prescription," I promised as my patient stood. "And, Becky, be sure to let me know if I can help in any other way. It sounds to me as if you've had a lot dumped on you."

When she answered, my old classmate still had that distant look. "Well, I'm seeing Dr. Lightfoot tomorrow, and if you don't mind, I'll ask her to give you a call. Maybe it would help if the three of us had the same baseline information."

Three days later, Dr. Elizabeth Lightfoot called. She was professional, efficient, and brusque. Noting that she was calling at Becky's request, she advised me that while our patient was making progress, she still had a long road in front of her. "After all, she's been seriously depressed since she was a schoolgirl, and you can't expect her to work her way out of that overnight."

"Since she was a schoolgirl?" I echoed. "I thought you were seeing her for the aftershocks of her parents' deaths."

Dr. Lightfoot cleared her throat. "That's exactly what Becky told me that you would think, Dr. Jenkins. That's the main reason why I'm calling. Ms. Bentham, who is one of the bravest people I have ever met, has really just started to deal with the effects of something that never fails to shock you small-town doctors—incest."

"Incest!"

Our conversation had developed a definite pattern. I was echoing everything that my colleague said.

Simple Gifts

"That's right, Doctor. Starting when Becky was thirteen years old and continuing until her stepfather's death last year. In our weekly visits, my main goal is to help her get a handle on the dynamics that quite possibly have destroyed forever her chances of living a reasonably normal life."

Now I was too stunned to even echo, and Dr. Lightfoot went on. "And there's another reason for my call, Dr. Jenkins. When Becky told me about your twelve years of school together, I suggested that she see you as her family physician. While she struggles with issue of reality, it may be beneficial if she works with someone who is acquainted with her background." Promising to call again, Dr. Lightfoot said that she was looking forward to working with me.

After noting that I was looking forward to working with her, I hung up the receiver and looked with raw disbelief at Becky's chart. Incest, that most ancient and unimaginable of all domestic crimes, had touched a friend of mine on Main Street.

We physicians are not very adept at identifying this form of child abuse. In spite of tremendous under-reporting, at least one hundred thousand cases of incest occur annually in the United States. At the core of each case report is a tragically confused child who has experienced the violation of multiple boundaries—physical, emotional, and spiritual. And now, taking my first look through this new lens, I thought about Becky and her family.

During our school days, Becky's mother had been a sickly person who rarely showed up for school plays and parties. When Becky was a third grader, her father had been electrocuted during a work accident. Her mother had emerged from her hypochondriasis only long enough to complete a period of public bereavement before marrying her second husband.

Becky's stepfather—a short balding insurance executive—seemed to be the ideal companion for his increasingly indisposed wife. Although he was a church elder, a Rotary Club officer, and an active PTA member, he never missed one of his stepdaughter's basketball games. Thinking about his seat on the front of the bleachers, I suddenly felt nauseated.

"So I'm relieved that you know all about it," Becky Bentham remarked when she showed up two months later for her next prescription refill.

I didn't share my patient's feelings. Like ripples on a pond, the widening influence of her stepfather's abuse had shaken my own innocence. No longer did I feel the same about the sturdy houses on Main Street.

Simple Gifts

My patient concurred with her psychologist's assessment that she was improving. During adolescence, Becky had suffered from recurrent insomnia that began with her stepfather's first nocturnal visit. As an eighth grader, Becky at first thought she was having nightmares. Sometimes she would awaken to find her mouth too dry to even whisper to the shadowy figure sitting on her bed. As the trap tightened, there had been no escape.

"I've often wondered how much Mother knew," Becky commented.

I shrugged. How could any household resident fail to sense, sometime in twenty-five years, the ghastliness of what was going on? But, on the other hand, Becky's mother for most of her life had struggled with an assortment of illnesses that, while often imaginary, had nevertheless been debilitating. Had this mother sacrificed her daughter on the crude altar of her own self-absorption?

As for Becky, she had always been certain that everything was her fault. Afraid to go to college, she had taken a job at the insurance company where her stepfather worked. In the daytime, the two of them commuted in the same car, and in the evenings, they cared for the invalid that bound them together. And during their nights, there was the same dark and well-kept secret. After her parents' funeral, Becky consulted a psychologist.

"Dr. Lightfoot tells me that you've made excellent progress," I said.

My patient's face brightened as she told me about university night classes and her planned degree in business administration. Already, she had enjoyed a work promotion and was sporting a new hairstyle.

Several months passed before the day of Becky's momentous announcement. "Dr. Jenkins, I'm going to miss seeing you. This will be my last appointment before I move."

My face registered my surprise.

"Lots of other people will be as astonished as you are," Becky assured me. The Main Street house had sold before the realtor's signs went up. A retired couple had snapped it up at the listed price. They had wanted an old-fashioned Southern house far away from the evils of the city.

"Congratulations!"

My patient's face was serious. "To get on with my life, I have to get away from that house."

I nodded.

"Dr. Lightfoot says that I'm doing the right thing. Somehow I just can't seem to make a clean break with the past and still live here in Madison. It's so hard to be honest with people that have known you all your life. So many times during the years, I've wanted to tell somebody, and people just won't let you."

I thought about the peculiarly blind conservatism of the small town, where the first and greatest commandment is that no occupant shall ever startle anyone else. With religious fervor, small-town citizens build graven images of one another and then destroy anyone who desecrates their shrine.

"So it's time to ditch the baggage and find some dreams." Becky's voice was wistful.

"You've worked hard on the baggage," I said, "and I'm sure that, somewhere out there, the dreams are waiting for you."

As my patient left, she was smiling through her tears.

CHAPTER TWENTY-THREE

MRS. MCALLISTER'S TOP PRIORITY

You can't learn too soon that the most useful thing about a principle is that it can always be sacrificed to expediency.
—W. Somerset Maugham, *The Circle*, 1921

"So how do you like the farmer on the checkout counter?" As Ellen tightened the polka-dot bow tie on a large stuffed bunny, she turned to me. Our new bunny, dressed in denim overalls, was clutching a rake and two packets of carrot seed.

"Oh, he's a fine fellow, indeed!" A gardener myself, I instantly liked the new arrival. I was still admiring his painted red smile when a slim teenaged girl walked through the door.

"I guess I'm a little early," she said hesitantly.

Assuring the attractive brunette that her timing was perfect, Ellen escorted her to an exam room and then returned to the checkout counter. "That's Patty McAllister, Dr. J."

"Should I know her?"

"Well, you certainly know her mother. Mona McAllister was one of the first people to see you last fall after the office opened. Mona adopted Patty when she was just a baby. I guess maybe that makes her a mother." Ellen's hazel eyes looked doubtful. "Mona's always been so completely fired up over stopping abortions that I wonder if she didn't consider Patty to be just one more pro-life project."

"Now I know who you're talking about. Mrs. McAllister came in with campaign literature during last year's elections."

As Ellen confirmed that I was remembering the right politician, I thought about a coiffured blonde sitting on a chair in the partially plastered space that was becoming my office. Her manicured hand—with hot pink fingernails that were color coordinates of a three-piece suit—had brushed the sawdust from the chair. Mrs. McAllister had come to educate the county's new doctor about the moral urgency of voting for her candidate.

"Her daughter doesn't look sick," I observed.

"I'm not sure why Patty's here. She called this morning from the high school pay phone and just said that it was something personal."

"Well, we'll know in a few minutes." Opening my top file drawer, I rummaged through half-a-dozen folders before I finally located Mrs. McAllister's election-year brochure.

Printed on quality white paper in red and blue ink, it summarized the many hazards of abortion. A boldface sentence caught my eye. "Every child is made in the image of God."

"Now what does that really mean?" I mused.

I was still wondering when Ellen handed me the new chart and told me that Patty's pregnancy test was positive.

I stared at the lab report. My patient was only seventeen. "How's she handling it?"

"I'm probably more upset than she is from the looks of things."

As I entered the exam room, I sensed too that my patient wasn't worried. Her blue eyes were calm.

"Your nurse already told me about my test result." Patty's voice was soft but even. "Of course, I was pretty sure that I was pregnant."

In her daughter's composure, I could see the influence of Mona McAllister. "This has to be a major event in your life."

"That's certainly true. It wasn't something that I had planned for my junior year."

In its fresh beauty, Patty's face was like an April trillium.

"So, Patty, how can I help you?"

My patient said that she had read several guidebooks on pregnancy and wanted me to refer her to an obstetrician. Thinking about the single local specialist who performed abortions, I mentioned that pregnancy offered more than one option.

When my patient shook her head, a ringlet of shining brown hair fell across the graceful line of her neck. "For me, there's only one choice. I believe just like Mother does—every child is a gift of God."

Patty's smile was enigmatic, like the mysterious smile of an early Renaissance Madonna. "And besides, I really love Frank, and we're both looking forward to being parents. Frank will be such a wonderful Daddy."

"Does your mother know about your pregnancy?" Somehow I was certain that I already knew the answer.

"No, she doesn't. Mother is such a busy person that she isn't home very often, you know. She's flying back this evening from a conference in Florida. I'll talk with her tonight."

Thinking about that upcoming bedtime story, I suggested that my patient consult with her parents before she called me with her preference of specialists. Patty promised to be back in touch within a week or two.

In human experience, few things are as revolutionary as the anticipated arrival of a baby. I was sure that I would be hearing from the McAllisters soon.

My prediction was fulfilled in less than twenty-four hours. Halfway through our Saturday morning, Ellen told me that Mona McAllister was coming in at the end of office hours.

"Okay," I said, making rapid peace with the Fate that predestines medical appointments. Certainly, it would be preferable to talk with the McAllisters today than to work them into a busy Monday.

When I walked into the exam room, I blinked. Like an equatorial sun, the formidable presence of Mona McAllister permeated every cranny and corner. Her husband—a lesser moon—inadequately reflected her solar glory.

In fact, the McAllisters offered a striking contrast. Mona looked ready to step behind the podium at a national convention. Her thick blond hair, with a hue that suggested art more than nature, was decorated with two mother-of-pearl combs. Ample amounts of mascara, powder, rouge, and lipstick covered her strong face. Complementing her cameo earrings, a double strand of pearls rested on the lace collar of a formal blue dress. Sitting stiffly in the armchair, she looked like a nineteenth century English duchess making an obligatory visit to some inconsequential colony.

The thin man introduced like an afterthought as "Mr. McAllister" was a foot taller than his wife and wore horn-rimmed glasses. Plastered over his prominent scalp were a few mouse-brown hairs. His swarthy skin and raspy cough suggested the prolonged use of cigarettes. A wrinkled brown suit hung from his gaunt frame, and his blue-veined hands looked as anemic as his personality.

Like a newly christened ship, Mona glided into our conversation. "Dr. Jenkins, I know that you're staying after your morning office hours, but unfortunately, I'm already overbooked for next week, so I needed to take care of Patty's little problem this weekend."

Returning her unblinking gaze, I felt that I needed the smoked glass that people use when viewing a solar eclipse. "Your daughter has already talked to you, then?"

In the background, the consort produced an apologetic half-cough, while Mrs. McAllister advised me that although she was disappointed, she was not really surprised. Her face—the face of a tigress—looked like it would rarely ever be surprised.

"When we have children," I countered, "nothing is ever entirely predictable."

"Patty's not really my daughter, you know. Of course, I adopted her when she was only six weeks old, and she's always had every advantage, but no matter what you do, heredity shows up in the end."

I felt a pang of sympathy for Patty. "This must be a difficult time for all of you."

Mr. McAllister escaped into a paroxysm of coughing, while his wife responded. "Patty has the same problem that all young people have nowadays. They're addicted to sex."

Glancing at Mr. McAllister's nicotine-stained fingernails, I noted that there had been a major shift in social values over the past few years.

"Real moral values never shift." Like the pope, Mona McAllister spoke *ex cathedra.* "We are living in a morally sick society, and its chief problem is just what I've already said—people are addicted to sex." She looked down at her manicured rose fingernails. "Sex is totally overrated in my opinion."

Beneath her unequivocal verdict was a subtle undercurrent. Could it be envy? I suggested that people sometimes enter into sexual relationships to try to find the love and security that they haven't encountered elsewhere.

Recognizing heresy when she heard it, Mrs. McAllister corrected me again. "To find real security, our young people need to get involved in the big moral struggles of our time, like the fight against abortion."

Simple Gifts

Security, maybe, I thought, *but what about love. Will they find that there?* Something in the McAllisters' marital dynamic hinted that during their years of doing the right things, they hadn't found too much of that scarce commodity.

As I opened the chart that rested on my knees, a red, white, and blue brochure fluttered to the floor.

"In a stressful time like this, Mrs. McAllister," I commented as I picked up the brochure, "it must be reassuring to know that Patty shares the pro-life values that are so important to you."

Mr. McAllister produced a staccato series of ineffective coughs. Behind her rouge, his wife may have been blushing, but it was impossible to be sure.

"Well, Doctor," Mona noted, "that's why we're here today. We need to come up with a quiet way to solve Patty's little problem."

As I tried to decipher Mrs. McAllister's innuendo, the brochure in my hand rustled as if it had a life of its own. "And how can I be of help to Patty?"

Like a fortune-teller studying tarot cards, Mrs. McAllister inspected her perfect fingernails. "Of course, I don't even like to say it, but Patty's much too young to be a mother. Really, Dr. Jenkins, she's just a child herself."

I struggled with rising disbelief. "So what do you think your daughter should do?"

"Patty will need to see a doctor who can solve her problem for her. She's too young to be pregnant."

I stared at Mona McAllister. "But I don't think that your daughter is interested in having an abortion."

Like a red flag in front of an eager Spanish bull, I waved that politicized word in front of the politician. This time, Mona was definitely flushing. Even her cosmetic exoskeleton could not completely camouflage her reaction.

Her reply caught me completely off guard. Instead of an emotional exclamation, it was a desiccated sentence from which all moist feelings had been thoroughly wrung out.

"No daughter of mine is going to have a baby by a black man," Mona announced. "In this world, there are some things that are worse than abortion, and in my book, that's one of them."

In my confusion, I glanced at Mr. McAllister. Cowering in the background, he looked desperate. Probably more than anything else, he needed an hour or two of uninterrupted chain-smoking.

When I looked down at the brochure, its Delphic message flashed back. "Every child is made in the image of God."

"Well, I'm surprised," I finally managed.

Mrs. McAllister's condescending smile was a blend of patrician superiority and political expediency. Only a moment ago, she had let me glimpse a Southern mother's feelings, but now she once again was a blue blood.

"So you may take care of it for us, Dr. Jenkins," she stated, as if concluding a mutually agreeable business deal. "I'm going to be gone next week, of course, but you can set up Patty's appointment for the following week. It's all very inconvenient, but I suppose that it can't be helped."

"And how does Patty feel about all this?"

Mona's eyes told me that my question was irrelevant. "Patty is just a child."

I looked at Mr. McAllister. "And how do you feel about it?"

"He feels the same way I do." Mona's flat assertion stabbed like a dagger into my attempted dialogue. "Both of us know what's right for our daughter."

Looking first at the duchess and then at her shadow, I said that I thought that Patty had already made her choice. I reminded them that under Virginia law, a pregnant teenager is an emancipated minor and doesn't need her parents' approval for medical decisions.

Mona's mascara outlined her alarm. "But Patty really can't be expected to understand why an abortion, as bad as it is, may be the only sensible solution right now." Her voice—no longer patrician—pleaded for my understanding.

Suddenly, I felt a wave of sympathy for the politician-mother. How tough it is for us parents to accept our children's allegiance to standards that we sometimes find convenient to discard.

"Mrs. McAllister, I don't think that Patty sees this situation like you do."

"But you will help me now, won't you?" Mona's arms reached out toward me. "If you talk to Patty, I think she might change her mind."

Something in my expression blew away the hope from the politician's face. I said that I would be glad to talk to Patty anytime, but that I wasn't

Simple Gifts

going to try to change her mind. I felt that she was perfectly capable of making a sound decision, and I planned to support her in every way that I could.

With amazing rapidity, Mrs. McAllister accomplished her transformation from supplicant back to duchess. "Well then, I'll just have to work it out some other way."

As she brushed by me, her shadow—avoiding my eyes—was close behind her. When he finally reached the waiting room, he bolted to the outdoors like a rabbit. Watching through the window, I saw in quick succession a pair of shaky hands, the flash of a lighter, and several quick puffs of blue smoke.

At the checkout counter, I watched the pink painted smile on Mrs. McAllister. Somehow it seemed about as real as the red painted smile on Farmer Bunny.

"Just send me the bill," said Mrs. McAllister to Ellen. "I'll take care of it when I get back in town. And I see that you're out of my pro-life pamphlets, so I'll drop off another box next week."

The front door closed, and a car motor faded into the distance.

Ellen glanced at me. "Dr. J., I can't imagine how much fun it was to be in a room with Mona all that time. Have you ever seen a politician who is so fixated on just one issue?"

"Oh, I think that her agenda has more than one issue." I was still trying to sort out the clash of priorities that I had just witnessed. "At least, it seems that way to me."

CHAPTER TWENTY-FOUR

THE PHOTOGRAPH CURE

> **The art of medicine consists of amusing the patient while Nature cures the disease.**
> —Voltaire

"Mr. Firkins, which one of your medical concerns should we talk about first?"

Addressed to the gray-haired gentleman on the exam table, my question was eminently reasonable. Before today's physical exam, he had completed a three-page health questionnaire to assist me in focusing on his areas of interest. After wading through Mr. Firkins's inventory, I discovered an attachment—six additional typewritten pages filled with his ongoing medical problems.

He had not always been ailing. Just one year before, when Mr. and Mrs. Firkins had retired and moved to Madison County, they had both felt quite healthy. Five months later, Mrs. Firkins died in her sleep. Her autopsy revealed a massive heart attack.

After this catastrophe, Mr. Firkins decided to continue living by his favorite trout stream. His daughter, an only child, lived ten hours away in Atlanta, and he saw no reason to move again.

But within the past year, there had been a disturbing decline in his usual robust health. A chorus of troubling symptoms had triggered multiple

Simple Gifts

medical investigations, all with inconclusive results. This labyrinthine process had led my patient to no definite endpoint.

His first symptom, chest pain, had been truly alarming. Six weeks after his wife's death, Mr. Firkins awoke one morning with chest discomfort and trouble breathing. At his family physician's office, all tests were normal, and for several weeks, his pain subsided. But after a particularly worrisome attack, Mr. Firkins called an ambulance. First in the emergency department and then on a cardiologist's treadmill, no abnormalities were discovered. Afterward, whenever he felt sharp twinges in his chest, Mr. Firkins chewed antacid tablets and wondered what was really going on.

After the chest pain came the headaches. One evening after dinner, Mr. Firkins was struck with a searing pain behind his left ear. His family doctor checked his reflexes—they were normal—and suggested a daily aspirin tablet. But a week later, while reading a medical column in his morning newspaper, Mr. Firkins learned that early morning headaches can be a warning sign of a brain tumor.

Fortunately, his CAT scan turned out to be normal. At least, the neurologist said that it was normal. But sometimes when his headache popped up in a new location, Mr. Firkins had his doubts. What if something sinister was going on—something with tentacles that was stretching and growing?

And then came more symptoms, and days filled with visits to the dermatologist, the ophthalmologist, the gastroenterologist, and the rheumatologist. Every doctor identified some minor problem that, while needing no treatment, required both an annual follow-up exam and an impressive bill.

"So, after seeing all these doctors, why do I still feel so tired?" complained my patient as I laid his bulging chart on the counter.

I asked if he was sleeping well. Mr. Firkins said that, before his wife's death, he had slept better, but each night, he still averaged seven hours. Now, however, when he got up in the morning, he felt worse than when he went to bed.

"I'm not taking any prescription medicines," my patient reported. "Maybe I just need a pill to pep me up."

I don't know, I thought. *Maybe zest for living can't be replaced like a spark plug in a lawn mower.*

After touching, prodding, and listening to his healthy appearing body, I joined the host of specialist colleagues who found no telltale fingerprints of medical demons. Mr. Firkins's examination was normal.

When Mr. Firkins raised his eyebrows, his male pattern baldness stretched out endlessly, like a Dakota prairie. "That's good, of course, but why do I feel so bad?"

I commented that, since his wife's death, his lifestyle must be very different. My patient's ambivalence shifted to suspicion.

"Now, Dr. Jenkins, you're a family doctor. Don't start talking like a psychiatrist."

Half seriously, I noted that psychiatry was the only medical specialty that hadn't already worked my patient over.

"Shrinks just aren't for me." Mr. Firkins's clinched fists were definite. At the University, he had completed a bereavement workshop and had disliked group therapy.

The energy in my patient's voice invited my next question. "Was anyone in your group taking an antidepressant?"

"Two ladies were." My patient studied me as if, after all, I might turn out to be a psychiatric wolf masquerading in the sheep's clothing of family practice. "But they both cried all the time, and I never do that."

After commenting that depression can affect individuals in different ways, I suggested that Mr. Firkins try an antidepressant to see if it would boost his energy level.

"Why, that's just what I said ten minutes ago, Doctor. I need a pep pill. Is that what you're going to give me?"

"Well, maybe you could view it that way." Thinking about how my pharmacology professor would rate my reply, I shuddered.

"Then, Doctor, I'm ready to try one!"

And after talking about how this type of medication works and about its possible side effects, I wrote my patient's first antidepressant prescription and wished him well.

But when he returned for his one-month follow-up, he really wasn't any better. Perhaps on an occasional day, he felt marginally improved, but not much more. I doubled his dosage and pointed him back to his quest.

When Mr. Firkins came into the office just before Christmas, he was openly discouraged. More tired than ever, he was planning to drive to Atlanta to visit his daughter. He was dreading the trip.

"Do you have any grandchildren, Mr. Firkins?"

Simple Gifts

"Just one—Andrew. He's four years old."

I commented that Andrew must be excited to have his grandfather coming for the holidays.

A half-smile crossed my patient's face. "Andrew's really growing up fast. I'll have to bring you a picture."

I said I would look forward to seeing one. Then after an esoteric talk about neuropharmacology, I wrote Mr. Firkins a prescription for a different antidepressant and sent him on his way.

On his next follow-up, Mr. Firkins reported that, in spite of a flare of his headaches, he had enjoyed his stay in Atlanta. "And here's that picture of Andrew."

I looked at a sandy-haired youngster standing in front of a lighted Christmas tree. In his arms was a snuggling ball of paws and fur—the golden retriever puppy that Grandpa had given him for Christmas.

"So when is Andrew bringing his new dog up for a visit to Madison?" I asked.

"In late March. He's really excited about being here during trout fishing season."

I smiled. Madison's mountain rivers—crystalline water cascading over granite boulders—are legendary haunts for both trout and fishermen. For the first time in three months, we didn't tinker with Mr. Firkins's antidepressant program.

Due to an intervening blizzard, my patient didn't return to the office until early March. As I walked into the exam room, he stood up and opened his wallet.

"What do you think of this picture?" he asked, handing me a snapshot. "This is Andrew's birthday party."

"Your grandson looks like he's having a great time." From afar, I admired the pure joys of youth. "If I remember correctly, he's coming to visit you soon."

Mr. Firkins confirmed that his family would arrive in two weeks. He had been quite busy preparing for their visit but overall felt better. He was looking forward to his daily pursuit of the elusive mountain trout.

We agreed to leave his medication alone.

April arrived, bringing with it another visit from Mr. Firkins. "Just take a look at these pictures, Doctor!" Several dozen prints covered the surface of my exam table. "Can you believe how much Andrew has grown!"

"His dog is growing too," I remarked as I scanned multiple photographs of Andrew with his fishing tackle and his golden retriever. In one scene, Andrew was wearing hip-high wader boots while he hopped across moss-covered rocks. In another one, he was measuring a shining rainbow trout.

"Sixteen inches!" enthused Mr. Firkins. "That's the champion catch of the week, and Andrew landed it all by himself!"

"With just a little help from you?" I asked.

My patient and I both laughed, and then he handed me a print of himself and his grandson, standing side by side and clutching their fishing poles.

"I want you to keep this picture, Doctor. I have another copy."

As my patient carefully picked up all of his pictures, I commented that he had enjoyed another good month.

"I certainly have." In fact, Mr. Firkins had enjoyed the recent get-together so much that he had already arranged a fishing trip to Atlanta over the upcoming Memorial Day weekend.

"I'm pleased." I reached for my prescription pad. "Certainly, there's no reason to change your medication when you're feeling so good."

Mr. Firkins meticulously replaced his photographs into a studio envelope. "Actually, Doctor, I won't need a prescription today. I stopped taking the antidepressant right after my last office visit."

"Oh really!" Pen in hand, I couldn't muster a more profound response.

Treating my irrelevance kindly, my patient assured me that he felt fine. If his old problems returned, he already had a month's supply of pills on hand, and he would start using them right away.

I looked at the man who, for the first time in a half-year of office visits, had not reported a single new symptom. "So when should we get back together?"

"Oh, I'll come back this fall for my annual exam. And if anything pops up before then, I'll see you earlier."

After Mr. Firkins left, I walked out to the front desk. As Ellen looked at me, admiration filled her hazel eyes.

"Dr. J., what new antidepressant did you prescribe for Mr. Firkins? It must be great stuff. Why, it's worked wonders. I can't believe how good he's looking!"

Reaching into my lab coat, I fingered my picture of two happy fishermen. "Ellen, I'm sorry that I'm not free to give you all the details, but we health professionals do have to be discreet. Patient confidentiality is so important, isn't it?"

CHAPTER TWENTY-FIVE

A MISER AND A LOVER

**Man's love is of man's life a thing apart;
'Tis woman's whole existence.**
—Lord Byron, *Don Juan*, 1818

"Mrs. Bryan, why did you wait so long to see me about your breast lump?"

As I looked at the thirty-six-year-old brunette sitting on the exam table, I felt a rising sense of dismay. I also felt frustrated. Under the blue paper drape was a hard disfigured breast that obviously had been abnormal for many months.

Before she replied, Maude Bryan's eyes told me that she already knew her diagnosis. "It started out like a sore, Doctor, and I thought it was just a pimple. None of the creams I've been using has helped, but I never felt any pain until last week."

When I had provided Mrs. Bryan with her first breast examination in five years, her left breast was much larger than her right. Actually, there was no discrete lump. Instead, the entire lower half of her breast had the texture and color of an orange—the classic *peau d'orange* sign that marks an especially lethal type of inoperable breast cancer. In her left axilla, multiple swollen lymph nodes were matted together in an inseparable thicket of invasive malignancy.

In the United States, 7 percent of all women sometime during their lives will develop breast cancer. Through the widespread use of mammograms and regular screening physical exams, most cases are detected early, and the outlook is generally favorable. As a physician, I had never before witnessed the dreaded orange peel that was underneath Mrs. Bryan's drape.

"Eugene has been working so hard to pay for his new bulldozer," she went on, trying to explain why she had delayed her evaluation. "He broke his arm last fall, and he's been trying to catch up with his work ever since then. I just couldn't stand the thought of handing him another medical bill."

This was Mrs. Bryan's first office visit, and as I thought about her medical future—brief and grim—I swallowed hard. With her advanced breast cancer, she could anticipate living for only a few more months, a time span that would be filled with the exorbitant medical costs that she had tried to avoid.

"You'll need to schedule an appointment with a surgeon," I said. Even with the undeniable presentation of metastatic breast cancer, a biopsy would be necessary to establish the diagnosis. From a pragmatic standpoint, its result would make no difference at all. For Mrs. Bryan, there were no promising treatment options.

"Make that appointment on a Tuesday afternoon, Doctor. My sister is off on Tuesdays, and she can go with me to the surgeon's office."

"Oh, I think your husband probably will want to go with you this time." I thought about the avalanche of bad news that was poised to crash down on these slim shoulders. Someone stronger should be with her to help carry the load.

"Oh, Eugene won't be able to go, Doctor. He can't afford to miss any more time from work. This is his busiest season. I'll be all right with my sister."

Ten days later, the surgical oncologist's consultation note confirmed my worst fears. Mrs. Bryan's breast tumor was an aggressive adenocarcinoma that had already spread not just to her axillary lymph nodes but also to her left lung and pleural cavity. For her own reasons, she had refused palliative radiation therapy. The oncologist projected a life expectancy of four months.

In fact, only six days passed before I received an urgent phone call. Mr. Eugene Bryan was insisting that I make an after-hours house call to check on his wife. She wasn't eating and was too weak to get out of bed. In his agitated summons, Mr. Bryan informed me that he already had missed two days from work.

As I drove up the winding gravel driveway toward the frame cottage, I passed a carefully tended vegetable garden. A dwarf boxwood hedge

Simple Gifts

surrounded the garden, and in the twilight, the white blossoms of the green peas competed with pink hollyhock spires for my attention.

Climbing out of my truck, I remembered that ten years earlier, the Bryans' only child had died at birth. On this remote hill was a pervasive—almost palpable—loneliness.

On the front porch, a stocky red-haired man was waiting for me. His ruddy face was covered with stubble, and his T-shirt was too short to cover his overhanging belly. Behind Mr. Bryan in the side yard were two yellow bulldozers and a sizable collection of earthmoving attachments.

"I want you to check Maude over this evening," he said abruptly. "I think she's going down faster than you doctors said she would."

Murmuring my regrets, I followed my host through a narrow low-ceilinged hallway leading to a small back bedroom. Illuminated by only one window and with no lamps in sight, the room was only a vague suggestion of space. At first, it was difficult to even see my patient. Certainly, her voice sounded weaker than it had been two weeks ago.

"This is a rough time for us to have a lot of sickness, Doctor," Mr. Bryan observed as my eyes searched for landmarks. "Doctors cost a lot of money nowadays. It isn't fair that just when a fellow is starting to get ahead, something always comes along to knock him back down."

"Hello, Mrs. Bryan," I said. Bumping into the edge of the bed, I had touched a thin hand. Maude Bryan's face was gaunt with dark shadows below her eyes. In just two weeks, my patient must have dropped fifteen pounds.

"Thank you for coming out to see me, Dr. Jenkins. I really didn't need you, but Eugene was worried and insisted on calling you."

"Certainly, I called him," Mr. Bryan interjected, shaking his head. "Something needs to be done. I can't afford to be a full-time nursemaid."

My patient assured me that the surgeon's pain pills were controlling her chest and arm discomfort. After taking two of them, she usually slept for several hours. At least for now, she didn't need any more medicine.

Mrs. Bryan's blood pressure and temperature were normal. Although her heart rate was a little fast, her lungs were clear. She told me that her breast looked the same, and I didn't recheck it. I hadn't forgotten how an orange peel looks.

When Mrs. Bryan sat up, she was so weak that both her husband and I had to assist her.

"So what are you eating and drinking now?" I asked. On the bedside table was a solitary glass of water and a straw. The bubbles in the water told me that it had been there for hours.

"Why, that's the whole problem, Doctor," Mr. Bryan declared. "She hasn't eaten anything since last week. She won't come out to the kitchen at mealtime, and she's only sipping a little water. She says that she doesn't want anything else."

"I'm drinking enough." Mrs. Bryan's reply was quiet but firm. "Eugene, you have enough other things to worry about without fussing over me."

"You're certainly right about that." Her husband's response was immediate. "It's a good thing your sister is coming tomorrow so I can start getting caught up on some of my bulldozer jobs."

Somewhere in the front of the house, a telephone jangled. Mr. Bryan walked slowly out of the room. "See what you can do for her, Doctor. We certainly don't need any more medical bills, but if we have to do something, well, then we'll just have to scrape by, somehow."

Along with his lumbering footsteps, some of the oppressiveness vanished from the back bedroom. For the first time, I noticed the pot of red geraniums on the windowsill. On the papered wall above the iron bed was a small crucifix.

"Mrs. Bryan, you need to be drinking something besides water," I said, looking at her bedside table. "Fruit juices would be good for you just now. They'll build up your strength."

Clutching her checkered quilt, my patient made no reply.

"And besides the fluids, you need to eat at least some solid food every day," I persisted. "Some meat loaf or tuna fish will give you the protein to keep your muscles working."

Again, I was met with silence.

"When your sister comes tomorrow, the first thing that she needs to do is to take some of your garden vegetables and cook up a big pot of soup. When you're sick, soup is one of the very best things."

Mrs. Bryan, looking first at me and then at the crucifix, shook her head. "I'm going to be all right, Doctor, but I won't need anything to eat. I've thought about everything, and this way is best."

Reaching behind her, I fluffed up her pillow. "Mrs. Bryan, my job now is to make you comfortable. What do you need me to do?"

Simple Gifts

My patient's weak grasp contrasted sharply with the determination in her voice. "Just try to keep Eugene from worrying so much, Doctor. I'm more concerned about him than I am about myself."

As I helped pull up her quilt, she patted my hand and promised to call me if she needed more medicine. She added that she probably had enough to last.

When I reached the front porch, Mr. Bryan was standing there, alone in the dusk. "Doctor, now, at least, you've seen it for yourself. Maude just isn't doing well. With all your expensive tests, you doctors don't seem to know very much about how fast cancer spreads."

Maybe not, I thought. *But we know volumes more about cancer than we do about a woman's love or a wife's willpower.*

"Certainly, she's losing ground more quickly than I would have predicted," I agreed.

"And, of course, the big medical bills are yet to roll in, aren't they? A few days in the hospital will wipe out a few months of my income."

"Mr. Bryan, if I were you, I wouldn't worry very much about that." After shaking his hand, I walked back to my truck and drove slowly past the kitchen garden and down the long driveway.

Three days later, a newspaper obituary told me that my prediction had been correct. After only a brief illness, Mrs. Maude C. Bryan, the devoted wife of Eugene F. Bryan, had died quietly at her home in Madison. In lieu of flowers, the family would appreciate donations to help pay her medical bills.

CHAPTER TWENTY-SIX

A MIDNIGHT CALLER

Midnight shakes the memory
As a madman shakes a dead geranium.
—T. S. Eliot, "Rhapsody on a Windy Night," 1917

"I'm tired of shelling peas."

My complaint was directed at Doreen, sitting across from me at our kitchen table. Of course, our predicament was entirely my fault. Three months earlier, snared by a glossy advertisement, I had ordered a new hybrid green pea. The garden catalog guaranteed that this one would out-produce all other varieties on the market.

For once, the sales pitch had been the simple truth. For days, we had harvested a bumper crop. But after three hours of shelling peas, I was ready to call it quits for the night.

All around my wife and me sat the fruit of our labors. On the table, a three-gallon aluminum bowl was piled high with peas. On the counter were stacks of plastic freezer boxes, tops, and labels. Beside my chair, pea pods overflowed from a bushel basket onto the floor.

A frugal housewife, Doreen hesitated. "We still have a peck to shell, and I hate to leave the kitchen in such a mess."

Encouraged by her ambivalence, I remarked that at 11:30 p.m., we weren't likely to have visitors and that in the morning, I would be glad to share the remaining peas with Ellen.

Simple Gifts

Doreen yawned and handed me a grocery bag. Delighted by our agreement, I put the surplus by the door where I would be sure to spot them in the morning. Only ten minutes later, we were sinking into a satisfying slumber.

My dreams were a pleasant collage—my childhood and the past week were woven together by the motif of green peas. Standing on her own front porch, my grandmother carried a red wicker basket filled with green peas. In her homemade sunbonnet, she was knocking steadily on the farmhouse door. Caressed by the peaceful narrative, I sank deeper into sleep.

Bang, bang, bang! For an elderly woman, Grandmamma certainly had a powerful knock. Opening my eyes, I suddenly realized that the pounding was not past but present. In fact, it was occurring at our own kitchen door. Springing from bed, I pulled on my slippers, tiptoed down the hall, and snapped on the lights.

The hall clock said that it was 12:30. After my hour of sleep, our kitchen looked like a battlefield where ignorant armies had clashed by night. Peas and pea pods covered the table, stovetop, and floor. In the chaos, the only sedate element was our cat, Oliver, whose blinking yellow eyes asked for some justification for my intrusion. As I walked over to the window, my slippers crunched on runaway pods.

When I saw the police cruiser in our driveway, my heart stood still.

Filled with dread, I unlocked the door and clicked on the porch light. Standing on our carport less than five feet away was a burly deputy sheriff in a brown uniform and a shiny badge.

"Good morning," I said, opening the door. My midnight visitor's face was impassive. I waited to hear about a fatal car accident or some other calamity.

"Doc," Deputy Pete Harris said, "I need your help."

In the fresh night air, I sniffed the whiskey before I saw my visitor's bloodshot eyes. As he stepped into the kitchen, I noticed his wrinkled uniform and the blue shirttail that floated along behind him. Only his weapon belt—with its nightstick, revolver, and ammunition clip—was in good order.

"What's going on?" I asked. As a local citizen, I had heard about Pete's tendency to drink on the job.

"I don't feel good, Doc." With one long arm, the deputy steadied himself against the doorframe.

I glanced down at my red striped pajamas. "Come sit down, Pete." I brushed a layer of pea pods off the closest chair. "Let's see what we need to do."

Wobbling on the threshold, my visitor winced and shaded his eyes. Away from the sanitizing night air, the aroma of whiskey quickly overwhelmed the natural fragrance of the peas.

Pete fumbled in his shirt pocket. "Gotta have a smoke, Doc." I didn't protest as he tore open a new pack of Marlboros. After a few puffs, acrid fumes swirled around our kitchen.

"Here," I said, pushing an aluminum measuring cup across the table. "Use this for an ashtray."

With a nod, Deputy Harris shook his cigarette in the general direction of the cup. His aim was off by about two inches, and a small dusting of gray ash, like the sediment from a miniature volcano, covered one yellow square of the tablecloth.

"So what's happening, Pete?" I asked again. Looking at my uniformed visitor, I was emerging from my panic. This midnight caller had arrived not as a public courier but as a man with a personal agenda.

Pete's reddened eyes looked at me through the simple sincere lens of acute alcohol intoxication. "Doc, I just can't get rid of this headache."

Against my ankles, something was warm and furry. When I looked down, Oliver purred and curled his tail around my pajama legs. In the middle of the night, it felt good to have an ally, even a four-legged one.

I asked my patient when his headache had begun.

The deputy dropped a cigarette butt onto the tile and crushed it with his steel-toed shoe. "Don't know, Doc. I've had it for a long time." The lighter's orange flame licked the virgin tip of another cigarette.

"Pete," I said firmly, "I think you've been drinking too much."

Given the assembled evidence, it was not an outstanding bit of medical detective work.

"I just drink to make my headaches go away." Through the thickening haze of tobacco smoke, my patient looked blearily at me. "This is one of the really bad ones."

"Pete," I said, "here's what we'll do. I'll get you something for your headache, and then you can go home and get some sleep." I studied the florid face bristling with gray stubble. "You'll feel better after a good night's sleep."

Simple Gifts

Walking over to the stove, I pushed aside a contingent of freezer boxes and turned a burner on high. As I filled the teakettle, Oliver waved his tail encouragingly. While the water heated, I checked my patient's blood pressure. To my complete surprise, it was normal. Against all the odds imposed by a self-destructive lifestyle, Pete's embattled arteries were holding their own.

"And who shall I call to take you home, Pete?" I dumped two heaping teaspoonfuls of coffee into a mug and added hot water. The jolting aroma of coffee competed with the cigarette smoke. "Shall I phone your wife or the sheriff?"

Alarm flashed across Pete's face. "Don't bother the sheriff. I guess you can just call Irene."

Brushing aside a pea pod, I placed his coffee on the table and turned to the wall telephone. After seven rings, a sleepy female voice offered a curt hello.

"Mrs. Harris," I said, "this is Dr. Jenkins, and I'm calling about your husband."

Irene gasped—her reaction to an after-midnight message was the same as mine. Assuring her that her husband was okay, I asked her to pick him up at my home.

"So what's he doing there?" In her middle-aged voice was both anger and relief. "He hasn't been in another accident, has he?"

"Not yet."

"Then I'll slip on some clothes and come right along."

"No need to dress up," I said tolerantly, looking down at my red-striped sleepwear.

While my patient sipped his coffee, I located our family aspirin bottle and shook two tablets into my hand. "Here, Pete," I said, handing him my secret home remedy. "Try these for your headache. They always work for me."

Without looking at the white tablets, Pete washed them down with a generous swallow of steaming coffee. By the time that headlights flashed in our driveway, my patient had finished a second mug of coffee and six more cigarettes and said that he was feeling better.

The woman striding across our carport wore a faded purple dress and a black sweater. Wisps of gray hair peeked haphazardly from underneath her knitted cap, and when she talked, her dentures wiggled. "Is Pete still doing okay, Doctor?"

Simple Gifts

I said that her husband was feeling better. Glancing doubtfully at my attire, Mrs. Harris stepped into our kitchen. As she headed toward her husband, pea pods crunched on the floor.

"Pete Harris!" his wife scolded. "Why can't you just stay home when you're drinking! You're not even on duty tonight!"

As my patient shrugged, his interrogator's eyes swept over the surrounding mayhem. Something about her thin lips bothered me. Perhaps she was only trying to keep her dentures in place, but somehow I sensed that she disapproved of our kitchen clutter.

"Pete, I think that I'd better get you out of here." Mrs. Harris's dress brushed against my garden basket, unleashing a small avalanche of pods. "It looks like Dr. Jenkins has plenty to do without having you on his hands."

Nodding my agreement, I slipped my arm under the deputy's elbow. Slowly and awkwardly, as if fighting off an attack of vertigo, my patient stood up.

"Do be careful, honey," Mrs. Harris cautioned. "It would be easy to slip on this floor."

Obediently, Pete looked down, and his weight shifted away from me.

"Careful," I said. "Don't lose your balance."

Agreeably overcorrecting, Pete lurched like a ship in agonal distress. Before I could yell at Oliver, it was all over.

The deputy's heavy frame stepped onto our cat, and the kitchen exploded with outraged yowls. Recoiling from the din, Pete collided with the bag of surplus peas, scattering them all over the floor.

Under the table, Oliver hissed at the singular outrages of this night.

Telling my patient not to worry about the cat, I steered him through ankle-deep pods and out onto the carport. As we walked to their car, Mrs. Harris told me that a friend had come with her to drive the cruiser back to town. I watched as she backed slowly out into the darkness of County Road 631.

It took the substitute driver longer to mobilize the cruiser. On entering our driveway, Pete had driven over three forsythia bushes, leaving his car in their botanical grip. When the cruiser finally drove away, an attached forsythia branch rhythmically thumped its way down the winding road.

When I walked back into the kitchen, Doreen was standing beside the table. She was yawning and in her hand was a metal dipper, half filled by cigarette ash. "I thought I heard Oliver fussing. What's going on?"

Simple Gifts

Gently depositing the dipper onto the mountain of unwashed dishes, I guided Doreen back to bed. In a few minutes, her regular breathing told me that she was once again fast asleep.

But as I looked at the ever-changing red numbers on my digital alarm clock, I was wide-awake. Only two hours before, I had been exhausted, but now I was wired. My head hosted a rebellious crowd of embryonic thoughts, all jostling for attention.

I thought about Grandmamma and her garden and the farmhouse. I thought about my bumper crop of hybrid peas and about my four children safe in their beds. I thought about Pete Harris and the tragic-comedy of alcoholism and about Irene and her midnight odyssey. And I thought about my own discontent.

Since my first day as a hometown doctor, my privacy had eroded like a beach in hurricane season. Pleased with my care, my patients followed me everywhere, day and night. Never was there a single hour that I could be sure was just for me.

Staring at the alarm clock, I realized that my midnight caller—completely unintentionally—had brought me a gift. For the first time I sensed that something was desperately wrong. It was something quite basic, but its name eluded me.

A barrier. Coming out of nowhere, the unexpected word was an exact fit. Pulling up my blanket, I repeated my new lullaby—*Barrier, barrier, barrier.*

And then I heard the soft footsteps of sleep and was lost in my dreams.

CHAPTER TWENTY-SEVEN
THE CHOCOLATE CAKE CURE

God and the Doctor we alike adore
But only when in danger, not before;
The danger o'er, both are alike requited,
God is forgotten, and the Doctor slighted.
—John Owen, *Epigrams*

"Blessed are they that mourn, for they shall have comfort."

The somber opening chorus of Brahms's *German Requiem* swelled over the packed audience at the Madison Choral Society's Spring Concert. Standing on the top riser with the six other bass singers, I felt a tingle with every note—the exuberance that marks the final performance of a major musical project.

"Lord, make me to know the measure of my days," the baritone soloist enjoined.

Reflecting on a week that had been crammed with rehearsals, I concluded that the measure of my own days had been full enough. I felt good. In another hour, I would be handing in my music and heading home. On this quiet Sunday evening in May, I planned to sit on the deck and watch the sun settle down behind the Blue Ridge.

Mesmerized by the conductor's baton, I hardly noticed the stir in the back of the church. Certainly, during the softest notes of the solo, one could hope for more respect from a dignified audience.

Simple Gifts

"Help! We need a doctor!"

An urgent male voice competed with and then completely vanquished the baritone singer. Gesturing uncertainly, the conductor raised his hand, glanced over his shoulder, and then lowered his baton. In the middle of an arpeggio, the string quartet abandoned their scores.

Tossing my music under the folding chair, I was elbowing my way through the tenor section when the demand resounded again through the hushed church. "We need a doctor back here. Right now!"

Pushing past a shell-shocked violinist, I raced down the side aisle toward the commotion. Clustered around a back pew, four or five well-dressed concertgoers hovered over a woman who was slumped on her side, her musical program still in her hand. Her face was pasty, and her lips moved inaudibly.

"I'm the doctor," I announced, stooping down to check my unanticipated patient. At her thin wrist was a rapid pulse.

"Marcella is having another heart attack," exclaimed a florid lady who was looking down at her stricken friend. "That's just how the last one hit her. She blacked out in the supermarket, and the paramedics had to shock her twice to get her heart started again!"

"Call the Rescue Squad!" I shouted, thinking about a defibrillation scene featuring fifty musicians and a cast of hundreds at Our Lady of the Blue Ridge Church. This afternoon, we had come together to celebrate a requiem mass, and now a selfless member of the audience had volunteered for the leading role.

"Take her back to the social hall," I instructed my fellow baritones who had dashed over to support their beleaguered colleague. In seconds, we had rushed the motionless body past dozens of distressed faces and had placed her on her back on the kitchen floor.

Close on our trail was my patient's red-faced companion, who came puffing through the door. Her musk perfume hung over the kitchen. "Poor Marcella! She's had another heart attack! The one she had six months ago nearly took her away, and I suppose that this one will finish her off."

Buoyed by this optimism, I quickly surveyed my patient. On her sweaty face was a puzzled expression. Over thirty seconds, her pulse rate did not change, and her breathing was deep and regular. When I touched her carotid arteries, she responded with a faint moan.

"Tell me what medications your friend takes," I said, glancing at the ruddy companion. Marcella, it turned out, took eight different medicines every day. Four of them were for her heart.

"And of course, she takes an insulin shot in the morning and in the evening." Adding this information as an afterthought, the friend shook her head. "Poor, dear Marcella. Heart disease is such an awful thing. Is there anything that can be done for her, Doctor?"

"Yes!" Leaping to my feet, I bounded over to the kitchen counter where our post-concert snacks—sealed in Tupperware and wrapped in aluminum foil—were waiting for us. Whipping off the lid from a promising cake box, I uncovered a three-layer chocolate creation, festooned with thick swirls of creamy icing.

Grabbing a serving spoon, I plunged it into the cake and knelt beside my patient.

"Marcella, I'm putting something under your tongue," I said. My patient's eyelids fluttered as I gently opened her mouth and inserted a glob of chocolate icing.

Glancing up, I witnessed the incredulity on the florid lady's face. In her small porcine eyes was a question. Was it not enough that her friend had been struck down by a massive heart attack? Why to this misfortune should be added the quackery of a local witch doctor?

"Bring me some ginger ale and a straw," I ordered. Looking squeamishly down at my patient, the violinist walked over to the refrigerator and filled a paper cup with ice and soda.

"Marcella, take a few sips of this drink," I said. Cradling her head in my left hand, I slipped the straw between her lips. With another moan, my patient began to drink.

"How long will it take the ambulance to get here?" The red-faced friend's question was addressed to everyone in the kitchen. "Poor Marcella really needs a cardiologist."

After learning that our volunteer rescue crew was still ten minutes away, the friend sighed and shook her silk hat sorrowfully. Over her ample bosom, she made the sign of the cross. She would wait a few minutes, she mourned, before telephoning Marcella's family.

Under my sweaty finger, Marcella's pulse was normalizing. It was becoming both less rapid and more forceful. As I spooned another heaping dose of chocolate icing into her mouth, she moved her right hand.

Simple Gifts

"I think she's coming around!" The surprise in the violinist's voice suggested that such an eventuality had never entered his artistic head. Lost in an opus that declares all flesh to be as grass, perhaps he had concluded that mortality is not only inevitable but also instantaneous.

Moving her head, Marcella stared at me through groggy eyes. "Where am I? What's going on?"

"I think you've had an insulin reaction," I said. "Your blood sugar dropped, and you blacked out."

With a nod, my patient swallowed more ginger ale. "I didn't take time for lunch today. We didn't want to be late for the concert."

"Poor Marcella just can't stand to be late for anything," her friend agreed. "She always says that it's so rude to walk into a concert after it's already started."

Intercepting our conductor's wry smile, I chuckled. Perhaps a little tardiness would be more forgivable than bringing the entire spring concert to a screeching halt.

"Well, Doc, what's happening?" The booming voice of Paramedic Rob Thorson rang through the church kitchen. Relieved to see him, I explained about my patient's acute hypoglycemia and her response to my makeshift treatment. Rob grinned as I pointed to the chocolate cake.

Soon, I was helping Rob to load our patient into the ambulance for her trip to the hospital. Although Marcella insisted that she wasn't feeling any chest discomfort, now was not the time to take a chance. With her medical history, she deserved several hours of cardiac monitoring.

After the ambulance eased away from the back door, I headed to the kitchen. I needed to call the emergency department doctor about the patient that was already en route. Waiting for the telephone, I listened as the florid friend briefed Marcella's relatives.

"Yes, it's really too bad. She's had another heart attack. She looks exactly like she did when we were in the supermarket that time. Yes, she's already on her way to the hospital. I heard the paramedics talking about EKG's and cardiac enzymes."

After a pause filled with sighs and with undulations of the silk hat, the friend concluded by noting that some supposed doctor who was actually at the church had tried to treat poor Marcella with a combination of chocolate cake and ginger ale. Fortunately, the bumbling clown hadn't really done any real damage, and the ambulance had arrived just in time.

Slinking into the back hall, I felt a hot flush from my neck to the roots of my hair. Oh, how sharper than a serpent's tooth is man's ingratitude!

When the conductor raised his baton, he focused on the bass section. Something in his expression warned me that he expected no further disruptions—lifesaving or otherwise—on my part.

"How lovely is thy dwelling place, O Lord of Hosts," I dutifully responded.

It is truly lovely, I thought as I listened to Brahms and watched the sunlight filter through the multicolored rose window. *Certainly, it is a lovely dwelling place.*

But it is not, I decided, *a particularly good place for a doctor who needs to treat acute hypoglycemia. Thank goodness for a conveniently placed chocolate cake!*

CHAPTER TWENTY-EIGHT

PUBLIC RELATIONS, HERE I COME!

All you need in this life is ignorance and confidence, and then success is sure.
—Mark Twain, letter to Mrs. Foote, 1887

"My, it's blistering out here!" As I walked beside Ellen toward the Madison Middle School gymnasium, it was easy to believe that the current heat wave had broken all the records. Scorched by a relentless sun, the sticky asphalt smelled like a tar pit.

This August day would see my first major public relations project in my hometown. Closing the office at 2:00 p.m., Ellen and I planned to provide free physical exams for seventh and eighth grade soccer players. Thinking about my civic contribution, I felt especially bourgeois and noble.

"With fifty boys going out for soccer, I'm glad that the gym is air-conditioned," Ellen commented.

"*Fifty* boys?" I looked at my nurse in consternation. A week ago, Coach Moran, who directed Madison's soccer program, had estimated that I might see half that number.

"That's what the school secretary told me yesterday. Maybe they won't all show up."

Pushing through the gym's swinging doors, I knew immediately that something was wrong—something quite basic and fundamental. Instead of being refreshingly cool, the gym was even more suffocating than the motionless air outside.

"This is really awful!" Ellen checked the thermostat. It was set optimistically at seventy degrees, but the thermometer beside it on the wall told a sadder story—ninety-three.

"I'll check with the secretary and find out what the problem is," Ellen decided. "I'll be back in just a few minutes. We need to get organized before the onslaught."

As Ellen left on her troubleshooting mission, I looked around my makeshift office. When Coach Moran had enlisted my help, he had promised to be on hand to assist me, but today he was nowhere in sight.

Glancing at my watch, I decided not to wait for him. Lifting two cumbersome boxes of supplies out of my truck, I lugged them into the gym and pushed open the gray metal door marked "Boys Locker Room."

The stench of old tennis shoes and unwashed gym socks—incubated to ninety-three degrees—slapped me in the face. My satellite office was not going to be a penthouse suite.

After I had emptied the boxes, no assistants had appeared. Remembering Coach Moran's promise of a scale, two tables, and some gym mats, I took a look around.

I found the scale in the back hall. It was one of the cast-iron, made-to-last-forever varieties, and as I hauled it around the corner, it dropped with a thud on the cement floor. Stepping onto the platform, I anxiously slid the weights along the bar. In spite of its recent trauma, everything worked well.

The Masonite folding tables propped against the locker room wall looked very heavy. The wall clock warned me that there was only fifteen minutes until show time.

"So where is everybody?" I fretted. As I dragged the massive tables across the room, they scraped noisily against the floor, leaving irregular patterns in the thick dust. Straightening their rusty legs, I flipped them right side up. One of them collided with a bang against the scale.

It took longer to track down the gym mats. In a closet with a nonfunctioning light bulb, they were hiding behind a barricade of soccer nets and baseball bats. Working my way into the closet, I selected four of the least bedraggled specimens and dragged them out. Along the way, I knocked over three or four metal goal posts, and their hollow clanging echoed through the empty locker room.

Simple Gifts

Under glaring fluorescent lights, I fished up a grimy towel from an even grimier sink and wiped the cobwebs from the gym mats. Once upon a time, when the world was young, they had been royal blue. Over the intervening centuries, they had faded to a more republican color. I was flipping one of them onto my makeshift exam table when Ellen finally reappeared.

I was primed to ambush her about the unexpectedly long absence, but she beat me to the draw.

"Dr. J., how did you ever get so filthy in such a short time?"

I looked myself over—undoubtedly, I was a mess. My shirt was covered with cobwebs, and my khaki trousers were smudged and rumpled. Along my forearms flowed brown trickles of sweat, like the channels of a river delta. "So what about the air-conditioning?"

Ellen's report was not good. Overworked by the heat wave, the school's cooling system had died just before noon. The repairmen thought that it might be operational again by tomorrow.

"In the meantime, this is as cool as it's going to get, Dr. J." Ellen scowled as she scrubbed my shirt collar.

From the cement wall above us pealed a deafening electric bell. It was 3:00. Our fifty boys would be arriving any minute.

Reaching into her handbag, Ellen pulled out a sheaf of yellow paper. When I commented darkly about the abundant supply of forms, she suggested that possibly Coach Moran had been thoughtful enough to leave us a few extras.

"Just in case we mess up the first three hundred?" I glared at my coolly competent nurse. When I am overheated, I secrete surliness along with my sweat.

Ellen ignored my churlishness and stepped back for a better view. Inspecting my shirt, she shook her head and told me that the grit had become part of the fabric.

"Does that really matter right now?" I snapped.

In my professional experience, early teenage boys are not fastidious health-care consumers.

Ellen informed me that it certainly did matter and that she would go find me a lab coat. Within seconds, she was back with a coat—cut from heavy material and stiff with starch.

"It's too hot for that," I objected.

In her drive for a high-toned operation, Ellen was not prepared to brook any obstinacy. Sullenly, I pushed my arm through a creased sleeve.

"So why aren't you wearing a lab coat, Nurse Wonderful?" I glared at Ellen. If I was going to be roasted on a spit like a Christmas goose, then misery would enjoy its company.

"I don't need to wear one." Ellen was perky. "I didn't soil my uniform."

Under normal conditions, I can master primordial impulses as well as most other men, but in this smelly sweatbox, my hands ached for Ellen's neck.

By sauntering into the locker room just at the critical moment, a pair of adolescent males saved my nurse from strangulation.

"Is this where we get our free soccer physicals?"

My homicidal urges thwarted, I acknowledged that it was.

Calmly unaware that she had been spared, Ellen directed the boys first to the scales and then to the bathroom to produce urine samples. Like God before the world began, my nurse had discovered a formless void; in its place, she had created a workable, if imperfect, system. Soon, our soccer physical assembly line was humming along like a well-oiled machine.

Except, of course, it was the people and not the machines that were well oiled. While most students wore only shorts and T-shirts, even this scanty attire was soaked with sweat. Like a runaway skater, my stethoscope slid wildly on a series of slippery chests, and my dripping fingers smudged most of the yellow forms.

All the urine samples were impressively concentrated. During a drought, the human kidney is the ultimate miser.

"You look hot," observed one thirteen-year-old, destined to be a rocket scientist. His damp sticky thighs adhered like plastic wrap to the even stickier surface of the gym mat. Nodding at his insight, I ran my finger down his medical history checklist.

"Are you feeling okay today, Reginald?"

"Nope, I'm half cooked."

My inspection confirmed his diagnosis. Although all organic systems were operational, he was dripping with perspiration. When he dropped his shorts for the time-honored hernia check, his underwear was soaked.

Reginald had no hernias, and as he pulled up his shorts, he announced that he needed a drink.

"Me, too," I agreed. My tongue tasted like it had been in a sandstorm. Leaning against the wall, three more soccer players shuffled their feet.

They could wait, I decided. After all, I should be able to work faster after a nice cold drink.

Following my guide to a wall-mounted porcelain fountain, I watched a bubble of water rise feebly to a maximum height of four millimeters. The subsequent trickle followed an irregular streak of orange rust into a grate that had not been scrubbed in my lifetime.

"You have to put your mouth right down on it." Demonstrating the proper technique, Reginald sucked the faucet like a lollipop. Recalling the families of bacteria that swarmed daily under my stethoscope, I thought about the awesome microbiology of this particular watering hole.

At a crucial crossroads in life, I made my choice. Better to die quickly from dehydration than to be eaten alive by an army of microbes.

"I have to get back to work," I said.

Looking puzzled, Reginald shrugged and walked back with me to the assembly line.

"There you are!" Ellen was as fresh and vibrant as ever. "We've examined twenty-eight boys so far, and it looks like another twenty or so are sitting outside on the grass. They say that it's cooler out there."

"Twenty more?" I licked my parched lips.

"At least. Of course, a few more may come along later."

As I beckoned to the next soccer player, I reminded myself that this was a praiseworthy public relations project, that I was a civic minded physician, and that I was dying for a good cause.

And so my afternoon in the Sahara dragged along. Like a nomad camel driver, I herded my patients through their exams, signed their forms, and then herded them back into the gym. Not allowing myself to speculate about how many more might be waiting outside, I pushed blindly ahead, sustaining myself with fantasies that were cool and wet—iced tea, snow flurries, swimming pools, mountain streams.

When Coach Moran walked in, he seemed like just another part of my mirage.

"Well, you've seen them all, Doctor Jenkins—all fifty-six of them."

As I grasped the coach's hand, I hoped that my grip was stronger that it seemed. I felt like a wilting pansy.

Elated by the thick stack of completed yellow forms, Coach Moran didn't seem to notice. "And I'm really sorry about the air-conditioning, Doctor. It must have been pretty warm in here."

For the second time in a single afternoon, I was seized with the urge to kill. Had I possessed the strength, I would have at least taken a swing at the smiling man who would rate Hell as "pretty warm." Wiping off a layer of sweat, I said that it hadn't been so bad.

When Ellen and I escaped from the gym, I drove straight back to the office and made a beeline for the refrigerator. Grabbing the pitcher of iced tea, I filled a sixteen-ounce tumbler and drained it in one long glorious gulp.

As my nurse sipped on her iced water, she fingered her lustrous curls. Not one hair was out of place. "I thought that today went well, Dr. J. This is a really good thing for Madison. So when's our next public relations outing?"

I emptied the rest of the iced tea into the tumbler. "Over my dead body! I'll never sign up to do another set of soccer physicals."

I drained my glass. "Well, at least not right away. Ask me again in February."

CHAPTER TWENTY-NINE

A DAY IN THE LIFE OF A MEDICAL MOVIE STAR

Every man has a lurking wish to appear considerable in his native place.
—Samuel Johnson, letter to Joshua Reynolds, 1771

―――

"Welcome to Madison's Taste of the Mountains!" Suspended over North Main Street, the three-foot high banner rippled in the September breeze. Today's street festival was the Chamber of Commerce's annual tourist extravaganza, when the town's population of four hundred souls swells to four thousand.

"It's a perfect afternoon," Doreen commented as I drove slowly along, searching for a parking space. On any other day, our tree-lined streets are half-empty, but today was not just another day. An ocean of cars had flooded the parking lot at the Farmers' Cooperative and had spilled over into the adjacent cow pasture.

"Maybe I should loop around and try to park on South Main," I said as I spotted the upcoming traffic barricade. A car horn honked, and I pulled to the side of the road to make room for the line of cars piling up behind my truck.

"Oh, let me do that," Doreen offered, waving to a friendly passerby. "Why don't you get out here and walk down Main Street? I already saw most of the booths on this side of town while you were at the office. I'll drive around the bypass and then walk up South Main to check out the photography exhibit. We'll meet in the middle at our church bazaar."

Behind us, the driver of a maroon van with Maryland tags sat on his horn. Agreeing to Doreen's plan, I jumped out onto the sidewalk. "See you at the Methodist bazaar at four o'clock!"

Doreen pulled away, followed by the burly van driver who scowled at me. I merged into the pedestrian stream that was flowing down North Main toward the center of town.

What an interesting assortment of people, I thought, looking at the pilgrims all around me. Just ahead, a young father with a toddler strapped to his back was hanging onto two more children. Behind me, three silver-haired matrons clucked about the homemade bluebird houses that they had just purchased. Now they were planning their assault on the antique stores.

"Wasn't that barbecued chicken the best you've ever tasted?" remarked one of the antiquarians.

Ever vigilant, my ears perked up. After a full morning in the office, I had dashed off to meet Doreen without taking time for lunch.

"Everything at that Umstadler booth is delicious," her companion agreed. "Before we leave this afternoon, I'd like another piece of that blackberry pie."

So would I, I thought, drooling over the prospect of a visit to my favorite local restaurant.

In front of me, a little girl tugged on her father's arm. "Daddy, I want some lemonade!" The family of four stopped by a canary-yellow canopy that shaded two glass tanks. Spraying upward in each tank was a geyser of lemonade.

A cold drink will be nice, I decided, lining up behind the children. Soon we were all strolling down the street, sipping on freshly squeezed lemonade.

"Dr. Jenkins!" A friendly voiced boomed across the street. Rob Thorson, Madison's star paramedic, waved from the Madison Rescue Squad awning. In his coveralls and matching baseball cap, Rob was a jolly orange giant.

"Doc, you need a cheeseburger to go with that lemonade," he advised. Raising no resistance, I soon was sitting on a lawn chair talking to Rob and munching through a juicy grilled burger that was covered with cheese, onions, and pickles.

Simple Gifts

"My, this is good, Rob!"

The giant grinned at my compliment. "Have another one, Doc. I know how careful you are with your low fat diet."

"Not now, maybe later." My decision had nothing to do with cholesterol—I had set my sights on a blueberry pie.

"Then you need a new hat." Rob selected a blue and orange baseball cap and crammed it onto my head. "There! That one is just your size."

After settling my account with the Rescue Squad, I headed back into the street. The sidewalks were jammed with talkative, laughing people—people who slapped me on the back with one hand while balancing a double-dip ice cream cone in the other. Loyal to the blackberry pie, I made a narrow escape from the ice cream vendor.

But at the Ruritan cookie table, I surrendered without a shot. I had already downed two large cookies—studded with chunks of chocolate—and was shoveling a dozen more into a bag when someone grabbed my arm.

"Why, if it isn't Dr. Jenkins!" I turned to see Mrs. Mattie Beasley, her gold tooth sparkling in the afternoon sun. Years ago, Mrs. Beasley had been my school cook, and over the past few months, she had become one of my favorite patients.

"Harold, you look wonderful!" Mrs. Beasley crushed me in her bear hug. "You've finally put on some weight, thank the good Lord. Life here in Madison is really agreeing with you."

I looked down at my bagful of cookies as Mrs. Beasley told me and everyone else how pleased she was with her new knee. Lifting her hemline, she pointed out the pink surgical scar that crossed her patella. Suddenly, she grabbed my hand and pirouetted around on the sidewalk. As my cap flew off, the appreciative Ruritans cheered and clapped.

"That's great about your knee, Mrs. Beasley," I said, dusting off my cap. "I'm glad that you're doing so well."

Clutching my cookies, I left Mrs. Beasley at the Ruritan table, where she was telling everyone in earshot about her favorite doctor. I blushed at her lavish testimonial.

Although the Methodist church was only three blocks away, it took me over two hours and well over $200 to get there. Along the way, I ran into dozens of festive patients and bought something from almost everybody.

From the Madison Historical Society, I purchased two shopping bags and promptly filled them up. There was a book on Civil War history from the Friends of the Library, hand-tooled sandals from the Lutheran Ladies

Simple Gifts

Society, a "Hike Shenandoah" sweatshirt from the high school ski club, three pairs of native quartz earrings from the Lions Club, two quarts of apple butter from the Wolftown Centennial Committee, and a cedar bluebird house from the 4-H Club.

"Dad, where on earth did you get that funky hat?" My son, Willis, greeted me as I touched down at the Boy Scouts' tent. At age sixteen, Willis had refined tastes in clothing that did not include an appreciation of my new baseball cap.

"Oh, from somebody down the street. You must have sold a lot of balloons today."

All around me, the Scout tent was filled with tanks of helium gas. Like ants swarming on an anthill, the Scouts inflated balloons and tied them with blue ribbons.

"Over seven hundred so far." The scoutmaster sounded mercenary.

"And you need one too, Dad," my son informed me, handing me a pumpkin-colored balloon. "This one matches your hat."

With a smile, the scoutmaster accepted my three crisp $1 bills and deposited them in a metal box that was already stuffed with the day's loot. I wished the Scouts a continued success, tied my balloon around my wrist, gathered up my shopping bags, and resumed my trek up North Main.

On the lawn in front of the courthouse, a battalion of parked wheelchairs gleamed in the sun. It was the delegation from Mountain View Nursing Home. From her wheelchair, another of my favorite patients hailed me.

"Haven't the Scouts sold a bunch of those balloons," commented Mrs. Mamie Marshall, smiling at my purchases.

I said that there was a huge crowd of people at the street festival.

"I know, Doctor. Of all the brooms we brought along this morning, we only have seven left." Mrs. Marshall glanced at a pile of brooms lying on the grass and smiled at me expectantly.

"Brooms?" I felt new respect for theories of social determinism.

"Our patient council makes them for a fundraising project." Mrs. Marshall selected a sturdy broom and held it up for me to inspect. "These are extra nice, Doctor. It's hard to find a really good broom, nowadays."

As I handed over the money, Mrs. Marshall beamed. Tucking her handiwork under my arm, I walked across the street toward the sounds of music. Underneath the watchful oversight of the Confederate Monument, the high school pep band was pumping out a lively program of Appalachian

Simple Gifts

folk music. Propping my broom against a magnolia tree, I sat down to enjoy the concert.

"Harold, it looks like you've bought almost as much stuff as my wife has." The man with the unredeemed Yankee accent was just behind me. Although his voice was familiar, I hadn't heard it in a long time, and now it was in the wrong place.

"How are you?" I said, twisting to face the speaker.

"It's been a long time," the distinguished man in the blue bowler hat said. As he slipped off his sunglasses, a tidal wave of confusion surged over me. Certainly, here under the Confederate Monument, this could not be my medical school professor, but then again, who else had that square jaw and those piercing eyes?

"Dr. Matheson!" I stared at my old professor. "Dr. Matheson!"

"Just call me Julian." My old mentor squeezed my hand and nudged the patrician lady sitting beside him. "Ellie, this is Dr. Harold Jenkins."

Mrs. Matheson's sunglasses hung on a silver chain around her neck. "It's a pleasure to meet you, Dr. Jenkins." She studied my baseball cap, balloon, and broom. "Julian has told me so many nice things about you."

I thought about the Dr. Matheson that had darkened my medical school years with his predictions of the inevitable demise of rural family practice. Looking at Mrs. Matheson, I swallowed hard.

"On our way up here this morning, I pointed out your office to Ellie," Dr. Matheson said. "That's a very nice building, Harold."

"And you must be very busy here in Madison," said Mrs. Matheson. "Your parking lot was full when we drove by."

"I do stay rather busy," I agreed, thinking about my first year of hometown practice. On most days, my office was overrun with patients.

"It's good to see a medical office thriving in one of our rural counties," Dr. Matheson continued. In a stylish athletic shoe, his right foot was keeping time with the bluegrass music. "Harold, I was just telling Ellie this morning that your type of practice is the wave of the future."

"Do you think so?" I asked. Suddenly, I felt dizzy.

"I certainly do," declared my professor, his jaw jutting. In his voice was all the infallibility that used to torment me.

Fighting disorientation, I invited the Mathesons to drop by my office on their next trip to Madison. After they jumped at the invitation, I gathered up my belongings and pushed on toward the bazaar. What a day this was turning out to be!

Simple Gifts

In the Methodist parking lot, under the shade of an enormous walnut tree, the ladies of the church were supervising a booming bazaar. Long tables sagged under grapevine wreaths, homemade jams and jellies, and freshly baked goodies of every description.

"Well, Harold, it looks like you've been shopping!" Fingering my broom, Aunt Lillian chuckled as she handed me a thick slice of lemon pound cake.

Leaving her post at the ham biscuit counter, my mother joined us. "So, did you pass up anything on your swing through town?" Her judgmental statement was softened by affection. "It doesn't look like you did."

With my mouth full of pound cake, I protested that I had walked right by the Umstadlers and their fresh blackberry pie. I didn't offer any explanation for my solitary blunder of the day.

"It's really hard to believe that you've been back home for only one year," Aunt Lillian commented. "Why, everybody's been talking about you today. You must be treating the entire county by now."

"So what did I tell you, son?" Smiling and shaking her head, my psychic mother headed back to the ham biscuit counter. *What a shame*, I thought, *that she isn't telling fortunes for the bazaar. She'd be a natural.*

"Hello, dear!" Doreen's voice floated through the mob of shoppers. "I know I'm late, dear. I'm sorry." My wife was so overloaded with packages that she didn't seem to notice mine. "Hasn't this been a wonderful day? I can't remember when I've had such a good time!"

Propping my broom against the walnut tree, I thought about the hundreds of friendly faces that had filled just one afternoon in my hometown—everybody from Rob Thorson to Mamie Marshall to Professor Matheson. Without warning, I scooped up Doreen, packages and all, and gave her a giant bear hug.

She squealed in delighted surprise, and Aunt Lillian laughed.

"I know just what you mean," I said. "It's been a day to remember—a day in the life of a medical movie star."

CHAPTER THIRTY

MR. WENGER'S LAST POEM

> The clouds that gather round the setting sun
> Do take a sober colouring from an eye
> That hath kept watch o'er man's mortality;
> Another race hath been, and other palms are won.
> —William Wordsworth, "Ode on Intimations of Immortality," 1806

"Here's another poem for you, Doctor." The serene glow in my elderly patient's eyes seemed inconsistent with his cardiologist's recent pronouncement. Mr. Seth Wenger was living on borrowed time.

I glanced at the lines of rhyming verse that, as always, had been painstakingly pecked out on an old manual typewriter. Over the years, the "g" key had worn down so that its imprint was now a mere suggestion of that particular consonant. "Oh, this is another poem about fishing, Mr. Wenger. You know that I always enjoy your fishing poems."

My patient chuckled. "Do you have time for me to read this one to you, Doctor?"

"Certainly."

One of the few life rules that I take seriously is to never miss an author reading from his own work. Settling down into the armchair, I handed the paper back to Mr. Wenger.

In a soft child-like voice, he presented today's offering.

> Fishing is one of the oldest of trades,
> Indulged in by young and old, by men and maids.
> It can be a sport or a source of food.
> Sometimes it's a failure, sometimes it's good.
> It depends on knowing where the fish are at,
> And having the right bait all down pat.

"You still go fishing every day, don't you, Mr. Wenger?"

With a kindly shake of his head, the retired Mennonite pastor corrected my theological faux pas. "Just six days a week, Doctor. The seventh day belongs to God, you know."

"Oh, yes, certainly."

Slipping my stethoscope under Mr. Wenger's homespun white shirt, I listened to the dysfunctional clamor of his heart valves. Damaged in childhood by a nearly lethal bout of rheumatic fever, all four of Mr. Wenger's valves muttered, hissed, and complained in a cacophony of pathology. Even with careful auscultation, it was impossible to be sure where the whoosh of aortic stenosis ended and the whistle of mitral insufficiency began.

"Does everything sound about the same in there, Doctor?"

After commenting that, in fact, it did, I drew blood to check the effectiveness of Mr. Wenger's blood thinner. Because of frequent medication changes initiated by his cardiologist, my patient was having his blood tested each week.

"Well, I'm ready to go home and head out to the pond." Slipping a pair of suspenders over his shoulders, Mr. Wenger fastened their snaps. "It's such a nice afternoon outside, Doctor—a perfect September day. It's too bad that you can't come along with me."

Mr. Wenger read the envy on my face. "Now don't let your patients make you work too hard. I've never been a doctor, but I was a minister for over forty years, and I know that everybody needs to have some time off. That's really why I took up fishing in the first place. None of my church members ever bothered to follow me all the way out to the pond."

As my patient rose slowly to his feet, I shook his hand and slipped his latest poem into my pocket. Inside my desk drawer was a sizable collection of this author's work. Today's manuscript would join its written companions.

On other office visits, Mr. Wenger had confided that his fishing excursions represented his chief source of relaxation. Living in full awareness of life's fragility, he could lose himself in the patterns of sunlight that dappled the surface of the pond. Across the back pasture field—comfortable in the company of frogs, turtles, and wood ducks—Mr. Wenger whiled away his passing hours.

Given the faithfulness of his treks to the pond, it was certainly fortunate that Mr. Wenger enjoyed his wife's fish recipes. On his most successful outings, he brought home bass, trout, and sunfish to share with his neighbors. And at night, after reading his well-worn Bible, he sat at his desk and composed poems.

"It's been another good week," my patient reported on his return visit. The nightly thunderstorms had brought the bluegill to the surface, and Mrs. Wenger had prepared her specialty—fish cakes seasoned with sage and scallions from their kitchen garden. When he described yesterday's feast, my patient's cheeks flushed with pleasure. Of course, because of some shortness of breath, it had taken more time to get to and from his fishing hole, but he had still visited it daily.

"I certainly hope that you didn't go on Sunday," I gasped. Mr. Wenger laughed at my tweaking of his religious habits.

"After church this past Sunday, I did write another poem." Under a pair of bushy gray eyebrows, blue eyes—the clear eyes of a young boy—looked out at me.

"Well, let's hear it."

Mr. Wenger unfolded a thin sheet of typing paper.

> The choice of baits for a sizable catch
> Is fish worms, mostly, even though bass will snatch
> Your bait and not even get caught,
> If you're not up to it as you ought.
> The best way to go about it, of course,
> Is to mind your own business—then you'll have no remorse.

"That's wonderful, Mr. Wenger."

Enjoying the afterglow of his smile, I listened to the ominous crackles at the bases of both lungs. Just as his cardiologist had predicted, my patient's congestive heart failure was gradually worsening. Instructing him to take an extra diuretic tablet each day, I watched as he walked down the hall, balancing himself on his cane.

The following week, Mr. Wenger reported that he had not gone fishing every day. On two different nights, his oxygen tank had not really helped his shortness of breath, and he had been too tired to venture outside. But, he noted, as his face brightened, he just this morning had caught three very nice bass.

"And so where's the poem for today?"

A wreath of happy wrinkles lit up the author's face. Occasionally stopping in midline to catch his breath, he shared his latest creation.

> Take a child fishing—he will always remember
> The joy that you gave from January through December.
> And it will help erase the generation gap,
> Teach the child perseverance and patience, perhaps.
> To sum it all up, it is well to know
> That fishing relieves stress and does good health bestow.

"It certainly seems to relieve your stress," I agreed.

Unfortunately, it was not bestowing health. Even with a boosted medication load, Mr. Wenger's heart was rumbling more ominously than ever. Again increasing his diuretic, I said that we would get back together in another week.

Two days before the scheduled appointment, Mr. Wenger's daughter called to tell me that my patient had died peacefully during the night. The family appreciated everything that I had done for their father. The wake would be at the Madison Mennonite Church tomorrow evening. The Wengers would be honored if I could come.

When I parked my truck beside the multitude of other cars at the church, I remembered Mr. Wenger's pride when he talked about his large family. His wallet had bulged with photographs of a growing tribe of grandchildren and great-grandchildren.

All of his family and most of his friends were at Mr. Wenger's wake. Through the long receiving line, dozens of friendly faces introduced me as "Grandpa's doctor." I smiled back at warm hospitable eyes that reminded me of Mr. Wenger.

At the end of the line was a petite woman sitting in a rocking chair. In a simply cut blue dress, she had covered her wavy white hair with a Mennonite prayer cap. Beside her, in a handmade pine coffin, lay the peaceful form of Mr. Wenger.

As I expressed my sympathy, Mrs. Wenger smiled. "Of course, we'll all miss him terribly. We were together for fifty-two years, you know."

I nodded.

Mrs. Wenger dabbed at her eyes with her handkerchief. "But if Heaven is anything like Seth was planning on, I expect that he's sitting up there somewhere by a quiet pond, pulling in one fish after another."

I chuckled at this novel view of the hereafter. Somehow, it was infinitely more attractive than the Methodist version with its classical harp concerts. "And no doubt, after his fishing trip, he'll sit down and write some more poetry."

Mrs. Wenger laughed. "Seth just loved to bring his poems to you, Doctor. Every week, he would be sure to have another one ready to read to you."

Inside, I felt a sudden unexpected pang. "I'm going to miss that a lot."

Mrs. Wenger reached into the pocket of her knitted gray sweater. "Well, Seth wrote this one for you last Sunday afternoon—he wanted to be ready to give it to you today." She smiled. "So, here it is."

Thanking her, I slipped the poem into my coat pocket. I wasn't ready to read it yet.

As I walked toward the door, a burly giant loomed in front of me. Looking out-of-character in his dark blue suit, Paramedic Rob Thorson was a one-man roadblock.

But even without his familiar orange coveralls, he was as jovial as ever. "Glad to see you here this evening, Doc. Wasn't Mr. Wenger just the bravest man you ever knew?"

Looking at the bearded paramedic, I didn't want to admit that I had never thought of Mr. Wenger as being especially courageous.

"He was a real man, Doc. I've taken him to the hospital any number of times, and when a man's that sick, you get to know him like he really is. And I can tell you that they don't come any tougher than Mr. Wenger. He was a velvet-covered brick."

Yes, he certainly was, I thought as I drove alone out of the churchyard. And how intensely was I going to miss this whimsical man—poet, priest, and fisherman. In the past year, I had come to know Mr. Wenger very well, and he was unlike any other man that I had ever met.

Certainly, with his genial optimism, he was nothing like my obsessed father. Thinking back to my father's funeral, I realized for the first time that I had felt nothing—no pang, no sense of loss, not one tear for a man I never really understood.

And Mr. Wenger's spirituality—idiosyncratic, understated, tolerant—was a very distant cousin of Mark Detamore's Baptist flamboyance.

Compared to the charismatic Mark, Mr. Wenger was less dogmatic and more real.

So why had it taken Rob Thorson to point out to me that, in a world of failed men, Mr. Wenger was so masculine? Surely, a trained medical doctor ought to be as skilled as a paramedic in recognizing manliness when he sees it.

Back at my office desk, I sat for a few minutes before unfolding the sheet of familiar typewritten script. In the silence of a deserted office, I read Mr. Wenger's last poem.

> If we could turn backward time in its flight,
> And we could again be a child for a night,
> It would never undo the things that are past,
> Nor would it stop time that is going so fast.
> But God in his wisdom has given us fishing,
> So rather than just lying around and wishing
> That we had more energy to use in the fight,
> We learn to enjoy the gifts of the sunlight.

Suddenly, my eyes were blurry, and I couldn't see the words. In my hands was my last remembrance from a man who had fought a good fight and had kept the faith. With clear goals and firm boundaries, he had touched the lives of everyone he met while always remaining true to his own unique mystery.

Pulling open my file drawer, I put my patient's last poem in its folder. Then I looked out the window at the dark shadows of the white pine trees and thanked Mr. Wenger for all of his simple gifts.

Edwards Brothers Malloy
Thorofare, NJ USA
March 10, 2016